MEDICAL DETECTIVE

MEDICAL DETECTIVE

Pascal James Imperato, M.D.

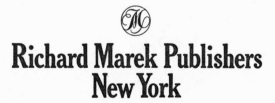

Richard Marek Publishers
New York

Certain names and events have been changed in order to protect the privacy of the individuals involved.

Library of Congress Cataloging in Publication Data

Imperato, Pascal James.
    Medical detective.

    Includes index.
    1. Imperato, Pascal James. 2. Epidemiologists—New York (City)—Biography. 3. Health-officers—New York (City)—Biography. I. Title.
RA424.5.148A35   614.4'092'4[B]   79-15315
ISBN 0-399-90058-6

Printed in the United States of America

012322

ACKNOWLEDGMENTS

I wish to extend my sincere appreciation to my colleagues in Kenya, Tanzania and Mali, to the staff of the New York City Department of Health and to my associates in the United States Public Health Service. Virginia Barber first put forth the idea for this book and I am grateful for her constant support, interest and guidance. My sincerest thanks go to Joyce Engelson for her invaluable assistance and editorial comments and to my brother Gerard A. Imperato for his useful suggestions. My fellow author, Errol Trzebinski of Mombasa, Kenya, was a great source of encouragement throughout the writing of this book and I am very thankful to her. And to my wife, Eleanor, who with good humor bore the solitude created by the writing of this book and who read and corrected numerous drafts with patience and a smile, goes my deep gratitude.

For My Wife
Eleanor
and My Daughter
Alison

Contents

MEDICAL DETECTIVE

CHAPTER 1

ZEBRAS AND HORSES

C-21 was a female ward at Kings County Hospital—a large room holding thirty-two beds and two smaller ones, each with eight beds. The interns and residents who ran the ward had their collective office in a small dingy room at the end of the corridor. The "main ward," as we called the big room, was bright and cheery. Several large windows and a southern exposure kept it filled with sunlight most of the day. But the office had only one window and it faced a brick wall. In the fall of 1960, I spent eight weeks on C-21 as a third-year medical student, doing my clerkship in medicine. Three of my classmates were with me on the ward and others were scattered throughout similar wards in Kings County Hospital and at outlying hospitals affiliated with our medical school, State University of New York, Downstate Medical Center.

The clerkship in medicine consisted of formal lectures delivered to us by various professors and intense exposure through the apprentice system to the diagnosis and treatment of a wide variety of diseases. C-21 as a medical ward in one of the largest public hospitals in the country was an ideal place to gather a lot of experience in a short period of time.

Once a month, the professors and chairman of the Department of Medicine came to C-21 to make what were called Grand Rounds. In medical jargon "rounds" means visiting patients in the hospital to assess their progress and evaluate the results of both diagnostic and therapeutic procedures. Doctors with patients in hospitals make rounds every day. Most medical centers and hospitals have Grand Rounds once a week. The format at Kings County was about the same as that used around the country. An interesting and often difficult case was presented to the chairman and to the other professors, interns, residents and students. Ward C-21's turn came around once a month.

The interns and residents tried to select cases which hadn't been in the hospital too long so as to cut down on the amount of preparation required, and if possible, they got a student to do the presenting. And no wonder. Whoever made the presentation had to memorize not only the medical case history and the results of the initial physical examination, but also the results of the tests performed on the patient and the patient's progress. The ritual which had evolved at Downstate and its affiliated hospitals required the presentation of all this information without reference to the patient's chart. There was no special value to the memorization of the facts; it was just part of the theater. The chart was usually held by the chief resident. He was someone in his third and final year of training after the internship and responsible for supervising the residents and interns. He stood next to the chairman, like a gentleman in waiting, ready to hand him the chart if he wanted it, but keeping it well out of the reach of the student. The only relief came from the interns and residents, who following the unwritten rule, stood near us and surreptitiously prompted us if we started to stumble—which we usually did.

Grand Rounds was a grand arena for upstaging . . . on the part of the professors.

In November of that year a sixty-three-year-old woman by the name of Etta Grundig was admitted to C-21 because of a three-day history of shortness of breath. Since it was my turn in the student rotation, I admitted her, taking a careful history and doing a thorough physical examination. All of this took me two hours and another two hours to record my findings on the chart. Actually the causes of shortness of breath in a sixty-three-year-old American female aren't numerous. I could easily have come up with what was the most likely diagnosis—chronic congestive heart failure. But I was inexperienced at the time and recorded a roster of esoteric conditions in my differential diagnosis. The differential diagnosis in any patient consists of a number of conditions which may give similar symptoms and signs. Making the final diagnosis involves eliminating the other possibilities by getting more facts from the patient, physical examination and laboratory studies.

Like most medical students, I had a natural tendency to hunt for the unusual first. In fact an important element in the training of medical students is to insist on their thinking of the common conditions in making the differential diagnosis. That goes against their grain since they usually feel that almost anybody can come up with common possibilities; they're interested in the rare conditions calling for extraordinary knowledge and intuition to diagnose.

Grand Rounds was due to take place on C-21 four days after Etta Grundig was admitted. But unfortunately, the patient who had been selected for presentation died the day Etta Grundig was admitted. The chief resident decided on the spur of the moment that I should present Etta Grundig.

There is an old saying that only fools go where angels fear to tread. I had apparently forgotten it in my delight at presenting my patient. I had already researched all of the exotic conditions I thought she had, or might have, or could have. Looking back, I expect that if she had had any of them, she would have died long before I ever met her. The residents and interns were amazed that I was so happy with the prospect of presenting on Grand Rounds. All of them dreaded it. I went home the day before, had a good night's sleep and arrived back on the ward early in the morning. When I did, I found the usual pre–Grand Rounds rituals underway. Mrs. Grundig was having her hair set in curlers by one of the nurses' aides and all of her bed linen had been changed. A change of linen had also been given to all of the other patients and the janitors were waxing the floors. Grand Rounds incorporated not only the concept of the chief assessing the knowledge of his subalterns, but also that of inspecting the physical premises. A finger pointed at a dirty night table was just as devastating to the residents and interns as the public revelation that they didn't know some trivial piece of medical information.

I knew enough to go over the history with Mrs. Grundig. "It's very important," I told her, "that you don't contradict what I say."

"Don't worry none about me, Doctor," she replied. "I'll keep my trap shut. You just wait and see."

15

At nine-thirty A.M. the interns, residents and students began filling the ward. You could distinguish them by the way they dressed. The residents wore white jackets and trousers and a white shirt and tie. The interns wore the same jackets and trousers, but white tunics instead of shirts, and the students wore street clothes except for a short white jacket. Next came the faculty, dressed in long white coats over their street clothes, and finally the chairman arrived with a retinue of gray eminences. The theater began.

I was beaming with self-confidence in the knowledge that I had read up on all of the exotic conditions I thought Mrs. Grundig might have. Here was an opportunity to show the chairman how bright I was. I positioned myself to the left of Mrs. Grundig's bed and from there could see Mrs. Viola Hudson, a sixty-year-old patient of mine who had been admitted for obesity and high blood pressure. I had told her about my presentation on Grand Rounds and she said, "I'll help you anyways I can."

"You may begin," the chairman said, ending the dead silence.

"This is the first Kings County Hospital admission of a sixty-three-year-old white female who came in with a chief complaint of shortness of breath," I began gradually.

"The patient's illness began three weeks ago when she noticed shortness of breath as she was hanging clothes out on the clothesline in her backyard in the New Lots section of Brooklyn."

The chairman unexpectedly interrupted. "Is that when it really started?" he asked Mrs. Grundig.

She looked at him for a brief second and then said, "Well, actually I felt a bit tuckered out when I was still getting them clothes out of the machine." Nodding her curled locks up and down, she added, "Yeah, it was while I was still down in the cellar. That's where I keep my washing machine."

I was afraid of this, I thought. He'll try to get her to contradict me.

I continued and gave her past medical history. "No history of operations, hospitalizations or serious illness," and then I went on and rattled off specifics with regard to each organ system of the body—heart, lungs, stomach, genital system, urinary tract and so forth. By the time I got finished with this, I felt punchy and must have been slouching because Mrs. Hudson made a sign with her two hands. It said, "Stand up straight and pull in your stomach."

16

Mrs. Grundig sat there taking it all in, smiling now and then at the thirty-odd physicians and students clustered around her bed in orderly rows of semicircles.

"You've never been sick before?" the chairman asked her.

I looked at Mrs. Grundig. She looked at me and then at the chairman. I held my breath.

"Well, come to think of it," she said slowly, "just once. I had typhoid fever when I was sixteen." Her sudden revelation stunned me. I wanted to drop through the floor out of sight.

"Typhoid fever?" the chairman exclaimed loudly. "Tell me more about it."

Mrs. Grundig went on methodically describing how she got typhoid fever in Providence, Rhode Island, how she felt, how her mother had treated it, none of which had she ever told me.

"How did you miss that?" hissed the intern standing behind me.

I hadn't missed it. During our whole two-hour interview, Mrs. Grundig had presented herself as a considerably healthy woman, now suddenly troubled by shortness of breath.

"Why didn't you obtain a history of typhoid fever in this patient?" snapped the chairman.

"My apologies, sir, but the patient did not give a history of the disease when I asked her."

"He's telling the truth," Mrs. Grundig blurted out. "I just forgot to tell him. You know how it is. You don't like to remember them unpleasant experiences, but all his questions the other day brought that fever back to mind."

I breathed a sigh of relief. Mrs. Grundig's confession rescued me from the chairman's wrath and from being ridiculed by my classmates, the interns and residents. It would have been a major failure on my part to have overlooked so serious a disease as typhoid fever.

After presenting my physical findings I went on to give my differential diagnosis, of which I was very proud. Looking back on it now, it reads like an index to a book on rare and uncommon diseases of mankind.

"The differential diagnosis is sarcoidosis, chronic asbestosis, silicosis, pulmonary paragonimiasis . . ."

"Stop! That's enough," the chairman said in a near shout. "What on earth ever made you think of all those diseases?"

17

"They are all causes of shortness of breath," I answered, and then I started describing the characteristics of sarcoidosis, intending to do the same for the other diseases on the list. Boy, this will really impress the chairman and the other professors, I thought, oblivious to the looks on their faces.

"Please stop, Dr. Imperato," the chairman said. Then he turned to the audience. "This patient has presented the classical symptoms and signs of mild congestive heart failure."

I was innocent enough to blurt out at this point, "I know, sir. That was the next diagnosis on my list."

"It should have been at the top of your list," the chairman snapped back angrily.

"Don't be too hard on him," Mrs. Grundig interjected. "I know he only looks like a schoolboy, but he talks like a specialist."

Laughter filled the ward.

"I don't want to have any of them diseases. They sound awful," she said pleadingly.

"Don't worry," the chairman reassured her, "you don't have any of them."

"Gentlemen," he said, "this is a good lesson for all of you. Always think of the common things first. Don't think of the rare and exotic conditions. Chances are they're not there. Remember," he said, turning to me, "when you hear hoofbeats, don't go to the window thinking you will see zebras. Think of horses. Do you get my point?" he added with emphasis.

"Yes, sir," I replied, seeing my brilliant diagnosis in shreds.

Think of horses and not zebras was the common slogan on all of the wards. In time I learned that the chairman brought out the idea in some way, shape or form every time he presided over a conference or at Grand Rounds. And time and again, students and interns came up with zebras. But as they moved into their residency years and gained more experience, the conditioning started to take effect. Finally, and much to the chairman's pleasure, they usually thought of horses and forgot the zebras.

Ironically, at that early stage of my training I had no way of knowing, nor did the chairman, that he was giving me the *wrong* advice. I was to enter a specialty in which I would have to think of zebras while other doctors thought of horses.

18

CHAPTER 2

THE WIND ILLNESS

In December of 1966, I arrived in the West African Republic of Mali, fresh out of my training as an epidemiologist from the Center for Disease Control (CDC) in Atlanta, Georgia. I was twenty-nine years old.

Epidemiologists are medical detectives, people who are trained to snoop out the hidden sources of disease outbreaks and epidemics and unravel the complex chain of events responsible for their spread. At the Center I acquired the basic skills of a disease sleuth and learned to think of "zebras" because more often than not these are responsible for the problems epidemiologists are called on to solve.

"You should be able to eradicate smallpox out there in a couple of years," my boss Dr. Norris said. I personally had my doubts.

"We're counting on you," he went on. "Mali has one of the highest incidence rates for smallpox in the world. Our success there is crucial to the worldwide eradication effort."

No one knew very much about smallpox in Mali, nor about smallpox in any of the other eighteen West African countries to which young CDC epidemiologists were being sent for two-year tours of duty. Worse still, perhaps, I didn't know anything about Mali. On the map of Africa it looked like a big chunk of the Sahara,

19

about the size of Alaska, but with the Niger River slicing through it in a broad arc.

It wasn't easy getting information on Mali, much less on its capital, Bamako, where I was going to be living for the next several years. Dr. Norris did tell me that Mali had a Marxist government.

"But," he added, "they're tolerant of Americans," a statement which didn't comfort me much.

When I eventually got to Mali what I found was a capsule of the past. It wasn't the Africa familiar to those who have been to Kenya. It was the Africa of yesterday, a primitive landlocked country of desert and heat, mountains and grasslands, a land whose life revolved around the Niger River, its swamps and flood plains. The five million people were very diverse, belonging to several different ethnic groups, espousing everything from indigenous religions to Islam and Christianity. They were farmers and herdsmen, nomads and fishermen. And they all had to be vaccinated if I were going to succeed.

The U.S. Government contributed one and a half million dollars to the vaccination program in Mali. We had twenty-four trucks to carry the mobile vaccination teams all over the country, as well as the smallpox vaccine, sixty-eight jet guns to administer it, measles vaccine for all children below six years of age, a warehouse full of spare parts, camping equipment, refrigerators and medical supplies. I was among the least expensive items.

I found that Mali's Marxist government and Malians in general weren't "tolerant" of Americans. They were downright hostile and went out of their way to harass the small American diplomatic community. The daily happenings of the Vietnam War gave Radio Mali and the local newspaper choice items for their steady barrage of anti-American propaganda. Diplomats have a high tolerance level for insult and invective, but I didn't. After I had been in Mali for a week, I decided that diplomatic relations should be broken immediately. Fortunately, I didn't share these thoughts with anyone else, and within six months, I had learned how to get my job done in spite of the hostility and harassments. Although I never became a diplomat, I grew tolerant. Not even the presence in Mali of two thousand Chinese and six hundred Russians impeded me as much as I had originally feared.

My job was to galvanize twenty-four mobile teams of vaccinators into an efficient work force, vaccinate the whole country, investigate all single cases and epidemics of smallpox, stop their spread and give advice and assistance to the Ministry of Health whenever they needed it. This wasn't going to be easy because the hospitals were staffed by Vietnamese, Russians and Chinese physicians and the Ministry of Health advised by Russians, Czechs, and a Frenchman. Thank God for the Frenchman, I thought. And I had reason to be thankful as subsequent events showed.

One day, just about the time I was getting settled in Mali, a ten-year-old girl named Jeneba Maiga stepped into a canoe with her aunt and uncle and sailed down the Niger River from their village, Titilan. They went eastward toward the great bend in the river, through a barren world of sand dunes and thorn trees. A hundred miles from Titilan, the Niger abruptly changes its course and flows southward. In this far-off eastern part of Mali, almost two hundred miles from the fabled town of Timbuktu, the Niger skirts the southern edge of the Sahara and then flows away from it. It glides past the straw villages of the Songhoi people and cool green marshes where herds of giraffe come to drink in the evening. There are crocodiles and hippopotami along this stretch of the river, herds of antelope, leopards and lions. Flocks of white egrets fly high against a cloudless blue sky and to the south of the river elephants wade through the shallow waters of Lake Niangaye and Lake Haribongo.

Jeneba's uncle was a prominent trader who sold salt and cloth in village markets downstream from Titilan. The salt comes from the mines at Taoudeni, in the heart of the Sahara, five hundred miles to the north of Timbuktu. It has been mined in large tombstone-shaped slabs since the sixteenth century and carried down to Timbuktu on camelback. Jeneba's uncle made regular trips upstream to Timbuktu where he purchased salt and cloth brought up from Bamako, Mali's capital.

Jeneba had sailed down this river before with her uncle and aunt, even before she had learned to walk. They made four trips a year, trading in villages along the way. But this time they were going to Tondibi, a hundred and fifty miles away. She had never traveled so great a distance before and felt a surge of excitement about being so far away from home.

Jeneba was one of many children. At an early age, her father,

21

seeing that his brother's wife couldn't have any children, gave her to them to raise as their own. This is a common practice in this part of Africa. Although Jeneba knew who her real parents were, she considered her aunt and uncle as her mother and father. She didn't see her real parents or her brothers and sisters very often, since they lived in Minkidi, a village forty miles upstream from Titilan.

Tondibi is a large trading center where the Niger meets the camel caravan route coming south out of the Tillemsi Valley and the dirt track coming north from the large town of Gao. The peoples of the desert, savanna and forest meet here beneath the straw stalls of the marketplace to barter their goods, exchange news and settle disputes. The Maure nomads bring dates and spices from the north; the Songhoi farmers, millet, corn, manioc and rice; and dapper city traders from the coast, transistor radios, flashlight batteries, mirrors and combs.

Jeneba found Tondibi an exciting place. The market bustled with activity and was full of heaps of spices, cloth, blankets, leather goods and gourds filled with milk, porridge and sour cream. Tradesmen sold pottery, basketware, jewelry and all sorts of foods, including millet cakes, peanuts, watermelons, dates and mangoes. Blacksmiths hammered out smart-looking swords from old truck springs, repaired hoes, sculpted wooden dolls for children and treated the sick with herbs and talismans. Next to them sat the leather workers, tanning hides, dying them brilliant green and red and stitching them into pouches, horse saddlebags, sword scabbards and wallets.

One afternoon, Jeneba's uncle took her to the edge of the marketplace. Stretching his arm out over the expanse of yellow sand and green thorn trees which ran down to the river he said, "This is where the Askia was defeated." She had heard about the invasion of the Moroccans. The Songhoi people along the river always talked about it. But now she stood on the spot where the great battle took place, where the Askia, the Emperor of the Songhoi Empire, sent out over thirty-five thousand men against four thousand invading Moroccans. Armed with firearms, the Moroccans easily defeated the Songhoi, who had only spears and bows and arrows.

Jeneba's uncle didn't take sides in his recounting of this story. He, like the rest of the Songhoi of today, is a descendant of both the conquerors and the conquered. And like most of the Songhoi,

22

he had only a vague knowledge of when all of these events took place. It was in 1591. But if Jeneba's uncle didn't know the date, he knew many of the details about the Moroccan invasion, details passed down through generations of minstrels and sung on quiet evenings up and down the river.

"El Mansur was the Shereif of Morocco," he told her as they slowly walked toward the river's edge. "He saw all of the gold coming north out of Songhoi and was jealous. So he sent armies across the desert four times and four times all of the men died. Then he sent an army out led by a man from a place called Granada. He had blue eyes and yellow hair."

Jeneba was spellbound. She had never heard these details of the story.

"This man's name was Jouder and half of his men were from a country of white people called Andalusia. They had been captured by the Shereif and forced to join his army."

By the time Jeneba and her uncle reached the river bank he had described the twenty-week desert crossing and Jouder's arrival on the Niger at Bamba. Jeneba knew Bamba and had been there just a few weeks before on their way to Tondibi. The rest of the story wasn't pleasant. The Songhoi Emperor or Askia, as he was called, was routed. Then Jouder took his army north and west to Timbuktu, conquered the city and destroyed all of the centers of learning. Another Moroccan army came down across the desert and Jouder was replaced by a cruel man because he was too kind to the Songhoi and because he told the Shereif the truth. There were no palaces of gold in Songhoi.

The Moroccan invasion of the Western Sudan, the area Mali now occupies, caused the total collapse of the Songhoi Empire and ended most of the literate civilization of this part of Africa. The learned men of Timbuktu were either executed or else sent into exile across the Sahara to Morocco. Few of them survived the desert crossing. In the anarchy which followed, trade and commerce died and the once flourishing trans-Saharan caravan routes and their numerous oases disappeared. Timbuktu was transformed from a rich entrepôt and center of learning into a squalid town of mud brick buildings whose inhabitants lived under successive conquerors. For the Moroccans were never able to consolidate their rule. Like many conquerors, they intermarried with the local population and were eventually conquered by successive waves of local chieftains and kings from among the Bambara, Tuareg, Peul and Mossi.

It was hard for Jeneba's father to come to terms with this part of the story because he was an Arma, a direct descendant of a Moroccan invader. His divided sympathies sprang from his own divided ancestry.

A few days after Jeneba and her uncle had been to the site of the Battle of Tondibi, she complained of a headache. Her uncle didn't think anything of it and told his wife, "Keep her in the courtyard out of the sun."

By the next day, the headache was worse, and on toward the afternoon, Jeneba developed a fever. Her uncle and aunt weren't alarmed because headaches and fevers are common complaints in children. They kept her on a straw mat in a cool corner of the courtyard. Another two days went by and although Jeneba's headache disappeared, the fever was worse. The following day, her uncle began to feel alarmed. He felt her head and thought, It should have gone by now.

He went to see the blacksmiths in the market and came home with some herbal brew reputed to be effective against fevers. It had a bitter taste and Jeneba didn't like drinking it. Her uncle hoped it would work.

The next day, Jeneba wasn't any better and her uncle began to suspect that her illness was due to some kind of curse. So he went to the mosque and asked the *imam*, a Moslem holy man, to come and see Jeneba. The old man looked at her, reflected and then recited a litany of Arabic incantations. "The illness will leave her," he said in soft comforting tones. Jeneba's uncle and aunt believed him.

But two days later, the fever was worse and then a peculiar rash appeared. Her uncle became frightened. Perhaps the spirits of the Songhoi killed by the Moroccans have put this curse on her, he thought. People rarely frequented the site of the battle, fearing the spirits of the dead.

I must get her away from here, her uncle thought, away from the spell of the angry ancestor spirits who live at Tondibi. He decided to leave Tondibi for Titilan the next day and scurried around clearing up his business affairs and making arrangements to hire a canoe with two paddlers.

Jeneba's uncle felt a sense of great relief as the canoe slid out into the main channel. They sailed upstream, against the current. But the oarsmen were young and strong and easily overcame the opposing current. The brown mud brick houses of Tondibi gradually grew smaller and finally withdrew into the flatness of the horizon. As they did so, Jeneba's uncle hoped that the spirits causing her illness would also withdraw and disappear from their lives.

The canoe made its way upstream for several more days. Jeneba's bumps turned into blisters which oozed a thick fluid which stuck to the blankets and attracted hundreds of flies. Her uncle and aunt drove the flies off by fanning Jeneba's body with a small piece of cloth. Some of the blisters were inside her mouth and she could hardly swallow even liquids. Jeneba drifted in and out of a semicoma, sometimes recognizing her uncle and aunt, sometimes not. They had never seen this kind of disease before, but they were positive that the spirits of Tondibi were responsible for it.

After passing the great bend in the Niger at Bourem, they came to the village of Baikana. The *imam* of the mosque here was renowned for his healing powers and Jeneba's uncle decided to visit him. He went ashore alone, leaving Jeneba with his wife and the two oarsmen.

"My daughter has been cursed by the spirits of Tondibi," he started off. The *imam* wanted to know what kind of illness it was, how long she had it, who had treated her. Then he said, "Bring her to my house."

The *imam* carefully examined Jeneba as she lay on a straw mat in one of the rooms leading off the large courtyard which formed the center of his living quarters.

"Was there a wind blowing the day you took her to the river's edge?" he asked Jeneba's uncle.

"Yes there was, but it wasn't very strong."

"Did it begin while you were standing on the site of the battle, or was it there when you arrived?"

Jeneba's father thought hard. He couldn't remember. The *imam* said it was very important. He thought and thought. Yes, he did remember. The breeze began after they arrived at the site of the battle, while he was telling Jeneba the story about the defeat of the Askia.

"Then it is as I think," the *imam* said. "The spirits have sent this illness out on the wind. You see," he said, pointing to Jeneba's rash, "only the wind can touch so many parts of someone's body at the same time."

"So it is a wind illness," Jeneba's father said to himself.

"But if we are so far from Tondibi, why has the disease continued?" he asked the *imam*.

"Some of the spirits have traveled with you in the canoe," came the confident reply.

The *imam* said that it would take him several days to drive out the spirits causing Jeneba's illness. He also had to drive the spirits out of the canoe.

"You are welcome to stay in my house," he said.

The *imam* wrote verses from the Koran on small bits of paper and had Jeneba's father take them to a leather worker who sewed them into small leather pouches. These were placed around Jeneba's neck and in the canoe. He wrote verses on a wooden tablet and then washed the ink off with water and had Jeneba drink the water. The magical verses would now be able to work against the spirits inside of Jeneba's body.

As the days went on, Jeneba grew worse in spite of all the *imam*'s treatments. Her uncle began to panic. He didn't doubt the *imam*'s word that Jeneba had a wind illness caused by the Tondibi spirits, but he was losing confidence in the old man's ability to heal her. The *imam* had to admit that he had never seen a disease like Jeneba's before, but he was certain of its cause.

Jeneba's uncle finally decided to leave and head home to Titilan. He thanked the *imam* and his family, who had done their best to care for Jeneba. Several of the *imam*'s grandchildren, who had kept Jeneba amused during the long hot hours of the day, came down to the shore to say good-bye.

They now set off for Titilan, three days upstream. The cycle of day and night passed and Jeneba grew worse. By the time they arrived in Titilan she was in coma. Her uncle summoned the *imam* and the blacksmiths. "It is a wind illness," they all said. But none of them had ever seen this kind of rash before. They all agreed though that the spirits of Tondibi had sent it out on the wind when Jeneba was standing on the battlefield. "Why did they do this?" her uncle asked, as he had asked the *imam* in Tondibi and the one in Baikana. The answer was always the same. "Only Allah knows."

26

Jeneba died a week after her arrival home. Her uncle and aunt were grief-stricken. She was their only child. The loss was overwhelming. In this part of Africa, death is accepted with stoicism and a compelling sense of fatalism but Jeneba's uncle and aunt did not react this way. They kept asking themselves "Why?" What had they done to anger these spirits. And why Jeneba? Why not them? There were no ready answers to any of these questions.

A week after Jeneba's death, the chief of Kandia, a village twenty miles downstream from Titilan, came to visit her uncle. He brought shocking news. "The two oarsmen who brought you from Tondibi have the wind illness."

"How can that be?" Jeneba's uncle exclaimed. "They weren't with us the day we visited the battleground."

"The spirits must have come up the river with you," the chief replied.

Three days later, word reached Titilan that the wind illness had also broken out in Baikana among the grandchildren of the *imam*. Panic and fear swept Titilan. What was but a curse on one child had now become a curse on all the people of the river. The *imam* made talismans for everyone and the elders of Titilan sacrificed goats and sheep to their own ancestor spirits who lived at the bottom of the river. A soothsayer and diviner was asked to come from nearby Minkidi. Every morning he went down to the river to implore the Tondibi spirits to leave. At the end of two weeks the soothsayer left, thinking his efforts successful. The wind illness hadn't appeared in Titilan.

Two days later, several children who had visited Jeneba complained of feeling sick with headaches. Then they developed fevers. Jeneba's uncle and aunt feared the worst. They knew this is how it began. Then the rashes appeared. There was no mistaking it. The wind illness had broken out in Titilan.

I was almost a thousand miles away in Bamako, Mali's capital, while all these events were taking place. The equipment and supplies for which I was to be responsible had been arriving by air and by sea and train via Dakar. Besides receiving it, I had to train a ragtag group of sixty-eight young men as vaccinators. I had to teach them how to use the automatic jet guns which can give a thousand injections an hour, how to repair them, how to vaccinate people and deal with possible medical reactions, and how to keep records. I myself had been taught these things only a few months before at

CDC; I was a professor a few paces ahead of his students. I did my teaching in the middle of a tin-roofed warehouse where the temperature was 100 degrees Fahrenheit most days. Outside it was 120 degrees Fahrenheit. I used to think that my whole body was going to drip away in perspiration into the floor.

My Malian counterpart should have been the director of Mobile Medical Services, but since this position was vacant I had to relate directly to the administrator of health. Dr. Traore was a roly-poly man devoid of the affability plump people are foolishly said to have. He was arrogant, pompous and patronizing, his vocabulary full of standard Marxist clichés. His bourgeois life habits made me think much of it was just lip service. I also knew that he had to be especially careful in dealing with me because I was the only American physician in the country. Mali's official anti-Americanism made individual Malians fearful of contacts with Americans. Dr. Traore went a step further. He tried to show a palpable hostility toward Americans; he wished openly to make life miserable for me. He succeeded.

In the first month I was there he prohibited me from entering all hospitals and from treating sick Malians. I swallowed this because the hospitals were staffed by physicians from Communist countries who would have refused even to talk to me. And treating these people held risks. I could be accused of making them worse or if they died of doing them in.

"You cannot travel out of Bamako, you know," he told me at one of our first meetings. I already knew that travel was restricted for Westerners in Mali. Anyone wanting to travel out of the capital and its immediate district had to submit a request in writing seven working days before to the Ministry of Foreign Affairs. Many were denied.

I can't direct a smallpox eradication program without going out to investigate epidemics, I thought. But I was willing to bide my time, assuming that eventually Dr. Traore would get used to me and then, I hoped, perceive me as neither threat nor scapegoat.

The wind illness spread among the eight hundred inhabitants of Titilan. Jeneba had returned there on February 18 and a month later sixteen people had the disease. The *imam* recited verses from the Koran, the blacksmiths administered herbal medicines and the soothsayer was called back from Minkidi. The disease continued.

28

Jeneba's uncle and aunt left Titilan for Timbuktu, over a hundred miles to the west. People clenched their fists in anger at them for having brought this disease into the village. Understandably, they feared for their safety.

The chief of Titilan finally decided to tell the commandant of the Cercle of Rharous, the administrative district in which Titilan is located. They were Songhoi and he a Bambara from a thousand miles away and they had to communicate through an interpreter. They didn't like the commandant because he wasn't one of them and yet he collected taxes on them and their livestock. As they saw it, he represented a distant government which took much but gave nothing in return. On his part, the commandant didn't especially like the Songhoi either, much less the godforsaken place they lived in to which he had been assigned. Not the best footing to begin with as far as controlling an epidemic was concerned.

There were no physicians in the area, but the commandant sent the *infirmier* (male nurse) who ran the dispensary at Rharous to Titilan. He was sincere and hard-working, but not much of a nurse. So when he arrived in Titilan, he looked around, saw thirty-odd people who had a rash and said, "They are probably insect bites." Not even the village children would accept that diagnosis and told the *infirmier* in local syntax, "You are incompetent!" He left in a huff, telling the commandant that it was nothing and to forget about it.

Boubarcar Ag Yusuf was a chief of the Kel Antessar Tuareg who camped each year a few miles downstream from Titilan. As was his custom, he made a courtesy call on the Songhoi chief of Titilan a few days after his arrival. As soon as he saw the wind illness he said, "It is smallpox."

Better-traveled than the villagers of Titilan, Boubarcar told them he had seen the disease several times among his own people, especially those who lived in nearby Niger and Algeria. There hadn't been any smallpox along this stretch of the Niger in several decades so no one alive had any memory of it. When the chief told Boubarcar what had happened with the *infirmier*, he was furious. "You are a proud people," he told the chief, "and your honor is your greatest treasure. You do not need this *infirmier* to stop the disease." As he remembered it, there were two ways the disease could be stopped. "You can get the vaccine the white people

29

make," he told the chief and the elders, "or you can make your own vaccine." This was a startling revelation to them, one they had never heard before.

The people of Titilan were not about to go back to the *infirmier*, so they asked Boubarcar to teach them how to vaccinate themselves. He did better than that. With the help of the blacksmiths of his clan, he himself launched a campaign against the disease by practicing variolation, although he didn't know that term. As far as he was concerned, he was vaccinating people in a fashion similar to what he had seen French doctors do in Algeria.

Variolation has been used for at least three thousand years and derives its name from the French word for smallpox variole. In this practice, the smallpox virus is taken from someone who has the disease and purposely injected into a healthy person. The rationale is that the person injected will develop a local skin reaction from the smallpox virus and build up an immunity which will protect against smallpox. Medical historians speculate that the practice started in China and among the Hindus and worked its way to the Middle East where Lady Mary Wortley Montague, the wife of the British ambassador in Constantinople, saw it in 1717. Lady Mary was intrigued by the practice, and when she returned to England in 1721, she had her daughter variolated. As is often true in science, several people made this discovery at about the same time. Lady Mary was not alone, but she exerted great influence as a proponent of variolation because of her close ties to the British royal family.

In America, Cotton Mather learned of variolation from his African slave Onisemus in 1716. He became a champion of variolation and popularized the practice in the American colonies, at a time when smallpox was a dreaded disease which killed half of those who got it. Even so, the practice of variolation has always been surrounded by fierce controversy. Not even Boubarcar, isolated from the modern world by thousands of miles of desert and wilderness, would escape this controversy.

Boubarcar had his blacksmiths variolate the people of Titilan. They used either thorns or chicken plumes and stuck them into the pustules of people who had mild cases of smallpox. They moved the thorns and plumes around inside of the pustules for a few seconds, and withdrawing the thick fluid, scratched it into the skins of healthy people. Boubarcar told the chief and elders of Titilan that most people would develop a small local skin reaction like the one that follows vaccination with modern smallpox vaccines. They understood what this meant since most of them had been vaccinated at some point in the past prior to independence. Young adults and children didn't know what vaccination was, but they accepted the word of their elders.

Boubarcar also knew that people who were variolated were afterward protected against smallpox. What he didn't know was that some people also develop smallpox from the practice. It all depends on the technique and a lot of other factors modern science still doesn't understand. But if the virus escapes from the local injection site and spreads through the bloodstream, then the person can develop smallpox. And worse, a healthy person without immunity can contract smallpox by coming into contact with someone's variolation reaction. The risk that variolation may actually cause smallpox is a major point in the angry debates which have raged since the days of Cotton Mather and Lady Mary. Confusing the picture still further is the wide variety of techniques once used. Some people crushed smallpox scabs into a powder and breathed it in through the nose. Others scratched smallpox scabs into the skin, some into a vein and so on.

The early proponents of variolation came into sharp conflict with the proponents of vaccination. In 1790, Edward Jenner discovered that cowpox, a disease of cows which often infected milkmaids, gave protection against smallpox. The milkmaids developed a few small sores on their hands which lasted a couple of weeks. After that they never got smallpox. Thus the expression "milkmaid's skin" came into use, referring to the clear complexions milkmaids had compared to the scarred faces many women had in those days as a result of smallpox.

Jenner and others popularized vaccination, as they called it. They took pus from cows with cowpox and injected it into people's skins. Those injected developed a local reaction and also immunity to smallpox. In later years, the vaccinia virus, a relative of the cowpox virus, was discovered and is used today in modern smallpox vaccines.

Modern smallpox vaccines were used in Africa prior to 1966. Of the liquid type, they were very often rendered impotent by the heat. Those vaccinated received no protection at all. Because Africans are splendid empirical observers, it didn't take them long to deduce that vaccination wasn't worth a damn. On the other hand, they saw that variolation gave them protection, or a milder case of smallpox if they did contract it later. It was natural, then, that the river villagers responded to Boubarcar's proposed treatment and made no further attempts to seek vaccine from the *infirmier* who had insulted them. What they didn't recognize was that some of the people variolated came down with serious cases of smallpox. But in such instances they concluded that these people had the wind illness caused by the Tondibi ancestor spirits.

It wasn't until mid-May that the commandant at Rharous heard what Boubarcar and the blacksmiths were doing. He had already begun to doubt what the *infirmier* had told him. So he went to Titilan himself and confronted Boubarcar.

"You had better let me inoculate you," Boubarcar told him, to the pleasure of the elders. "You've been exposed to a lot of people with smallpox."

The commandant had no response. He had never seen smallpox and didn't know what it looked like.

"But they're not insect bites," he said to himself. Then he visited Kandia and Baikana. The two oarsmen who had fallen ill in Kandia had recovered, but some of the *imam*'s grandchildren in Baikana had died. Smallpox, or whatever this disease was, was up and down a two-hundred-mile stretch of the Niger River. The commandant had been vaccinated once, but his wife and children hadn't. He panicked and dashed off a telegram to Bamako. It read in French: "Smallpox epidemic Titilan village stop disease spreading east and west along river stop send vaccine."

I wouldn't have known about the commandant's telegram if my friend and colleague, Dr. Jacques Dupont, hadn't told me. He had been in Mali since 1946, when it was the French Sudan. He started off as a French colonial medical officer in a remote bush post and eventually worked his way up to become director of Mobile Medical Services. When independence came in 1960, he stayed on as chief technical advisor to the minister of health to whom Dr. Traore reported. But the minister exercised little control over Dr. Traore and Dr. Dupont's position was correspondingly weakened.

In this case, Dr. Traore decided to send a thousand doses of Algerian-made liquid smallpox vaccine to the commandant by truck and boat, a trip that took three weeks. The live virus in liquid smallpox vaccines is extremely fragile. Exposure to even 70 degrees Fahrenheit for as little as an hour effectively kills it, rendering the vaccine useless. At that time liquid vaccines were of such limited value that they weren't even being produced anymore. Dr. Traore had some in storage which had been donated to Mali by Algeria two years before. This was the vaccine he decided to use, even though he knew that a million doses of a far more effective vaccine had been received from the United States.

The mass-vaccination program which I was to administer was to be launched after the rains finished in September. Meanwhile, the vaccinators and the jet guns were idle, and the million doses of vaccine were in storage. This American vaccine was of a new type that had been recently developed. It was dried and sealed in a vacuum in large bottles. In this "lyophilized" state the virus can survive very hot temperatures for weeks and warm temperatures for months. It was the development of this vaccine which enabled the World Health Organization to consider eradicating smallpox throughout the world, beginning in 1966. Lyophilized vaccines were ideal for vaccinating populations in the tropics where most smallpox cases were then found and where refrigeration was hard to come by.

When Dupont learned of Traore's decision to use the Algerian vaccine, he was enraged and requested an explanation.

"We can show that a sister socialist state is helping us," said the minister in reply to Dr. Dupont's protest, closing the issue.

"Not only is the vaccine probably impotent," said Dr. Dupont to me. "But Traore is sending a pathetically inadequate amount."

We both knew that the Cercle of Rharous had about seventy thousand people, most living along the river. All of them plus those living in the adjacent Cercles of Bourem and Timbuktu were potentially endangered. And yet we knew that six vaccinators using jet guns could vaccinate the whole population in less than two weeks and stop the epidemic. Politics dictated otherwise.

When I learned of the commandant's telegram, I went to see Dr. Traore. The meeting lasted for two hours. I wanted to fly to Timbuktu with six vaccinators, jet guns and a hundred thousand doses of heat-resistant vaccine. I was eager to investigate the epidemic, find out how severe the disease was, its rate of spread, its mortality

33

rate and all of the other characteristics we didn't know about small-pox in Africa.

"Your help isn't needed," Traore said with an arrogant wave of his arm. "The local administrative and medical authorities have the situation under control."

I had no way of knowing who those authorities were.

"Besides," he added, "it's over two hundred kilometers from Timbuktu to the villages where the disease is present and the track is very bad."

That didn't discourage me. "I don't mind bad tracks," I said.

"Unfortunately, there is no transport available for you in Tim-buktu. The chief medical officer there had a Land-Rover but it broke down several months ago. Besides, he's in the Soviet Union for medical treatment and it would be an insult to him for you to go there without him being present."

The discussion dragged on and I got nowhere. He wouldn't give me the authorization to go. Dr. Dupont's efforts on my behalf with the minister had no effect. The minister deferred to Dr. Traore's judgment. But I didn't give up. For the next two months I tried to go to Titilan, but my efforts were in vain.

Then in mid-July, two months after the commandant's telegram, Dr. Traore suddenly called me to his office. Much to my surprise he agreed to let me go to Titilan. I was tremendously excited at the prospect of going, but baffled and troubled by Traore's complete change of heart. Later I realized he had no choice but to let me go. The epidemic was out of hand, and ultimately he would be held responsible for failing to control it.

CHAPTER 3

THE DISEASE THAT BEHAVED DIFFERENTLY

The Air Mali DC-3 made its way down slowly and cautiously through the choppy layers of the hot atmosphere. We had left Bamako at five A.M., following the Niger River up into the vast northeastern stretches of Mali. For most of the four-hour flight I could see only the broad river, now in flood, and its deep green flood plains stretching north toward the yellow sands of the Sahara. Here and there were scattered island villages, small clusters of brown-colored rectangular buildings, so tightly packed that from the air they looked like they were tripping over one another. But it was the breathtaking sweep of this landscape which gave it the essence of majesty.

Here I was, on a small plane, approaching renowned Timbuktu, a city which people call "the mysterious," and yet my feelings of excitement had little to do with the place. For beyond Timbuktu lay my real challenge, an epidemic whose nature and magnitude I knew nothing about, an epidemic which I had to conquer.

There was only a handful of passengers on the plane, including an elderly American couple who had always dreamed of visiting Timbuktu. They were from San Diego, California, and had a son who was a physician in private practice in Los Angeles. They hadn't expected to come across a young American physician in a place like Mali and repeatedly asked me how I managed to survive. They were aghast at the thought of my going off two hundred miles beyond Timbuktu. I was pretty scared myself, but didn't tell them. As the plane made a final swing above the landing strip, I glanced eastward. I saw a world of river, swamp, sand dunes and thorn trees and sensed the fear of the unknown.

"Ça va," said the driver who had been sent out to pick me up. I only half heard him. The heat was unbelievable, all-enveloping to the point of distraction. And a muffled wind carried not just sand, but the unfamiliar voice of the desert daring me to a challenge.

The paved road from the airport suddenly stopped in the main square of Timbuktu. Beyond this point there was nothing but sand. I went to see the commandant of the Cercle of Timbuktu, whose office was in a Moorish-looking building on the main square. He told me that one of his drivers would take me later that afternoon to Ber, an administrative post some fifty miles east of Timbuktu. After an overnight stay, I could start on my way to Titilan. I wanted to leave right away, but the commandant cautioned against it, saying that the heat was already too intense for travel, even at ten in the morning!

I spent a few hours discovering Timbuktu for myself. My initial impressions were disappointing. It was a town of twelve thousand people, built of gray mud brick. It was all one mass of gray: gray mud huts, gray mosques, gray buildings, gray fort-like bastions, gray dust all over. I stepped into the shadowed archways of the Sankore mosque which offered a cool sanctuary from the sun. Two old men were dozing under the arches. It was all mud, the roof, the minaret, the walls and the arches. The floor was sand. "Was it here that interpretations of the Koran were discussed four hundred years ago?" I asked myself. Sankore was said to be a great center of learning. I found nothing in it that hadn't been there for centuries and yet I couldn't conjure up my former visions in this place. For from all accounts, Timbuktu is physically the same today as it was centuries ago. "So where is the veiled promise of grandeur?" I asked myself.

The streets were deserted and quiet, the marketplace subdued. How could this have been the great crossroads of gold and wisdom the Europeans dreamt of visiting and the Moroccans dreamt of conquering, I wondered. The city didn't beat with the pulse of a vibrant life. It was as if it were asleep and I thought that perhaps it had always been asleep. As I inspected and probed the winding streets I sensed a present which was standing still. There was no struggle here or sense of purpose. It seemed to me that Timbuktu was standing alone, neither proud nor humble. It was just there, barely surviving, yielding nothing because it had nothing to yield.

How wrong I was! I visited Timbuktu many times during the subsequent years I was in Mali and lived there for several weeks. It was then that I learned that the renown of the place is not in what is physically there, nor in what had once been there, but rather in what had taken place there. All of Timbuktu's centuries of history and civilization are preserved in a language much different from stone monuments, royal tombs, castles and palaces and great museums. But on my first trip, I, like most visitors, didn't understand this language. I didn't see the story of Timbuktu preserved in its present-day ethnic diversity, in oral traditions and ancient Arabic manuscripts. Nor did I understand how and why the Western world made Timbuktu synonymous with mystery and in so doing made it to be in thought what it never was in fact.

That afternoon, I started on my trip east. The track followed the river. It was the beginning of the rainy season and the high gold-colored sand dunes sprouted a faint green fuzz of new grass. The sky was a deep blue splashed with large dramatic puffs of white clouds which reflected off the river's surface. Here and there were isolated villages built of mud and grass and off on the horizons herds of antelope and giraffe and occasional lines of camels: an untouched corner of Africa. There was no monotony along this route since each turn in the track brought into view spectacular landscapes of shimmering green marshes, tall rugged mountains and deep valleys.

We arrived in Ber toward sunset. The air grew cool and carried the soft music of doves and the quiet voice of the desert. For one of the few times in my life, no mechanical sound reached my ears. It was a strange experience. And at night the clear atmosphere let through the light of a thousand stars. This was a world where man could come into close contact with the cosmos. I felt something eternal out there, something unexplainable; it was there; it did not hide, but the mystery remains.

I reached Gourma-Rharous the following afternoon. It lies on the southern bank of the river, and since the track is on the northern bank, the commandant had to come across to fetch me in a launch. Rharous, as it is commonly called, is a small village of about nine hundred people built high up on the river bank. Behind it are enormous sand dunes whose sands constantly drift down into the village, accumulating to a depth of two feet during some months. The commandant gave me a warm welcome. He had received a radio message from the Ministry of Health announcing my arrival and also one from the commandant in Timbuktu.

When we got to Rharous, the commandant showed me the vaccine he had received. It had expired the year before and the *infirmier* reported that very few people had developed a vaccination reaction from it. The vaccine had been used only in the village of Rharous since Traore had sent a thousand doses.

I started out for Titilan in the afternoon with a lot of trepidation. I had never seen a case of smallpox before in my life. Neither had any of the professors who had taught me in medical school, although some of the people who taught me at CDC had seen it in India. In theory I knew what smallpox was, how to diagnose it and how to handle it. But now that it was down the road in front of me, I wasn't so sure of myself.

Titilan was a total surprise. It was really a composite of three different settlements, one on the north bank of the river, another on the south and the third on an island in between. The settlement on the north bank was a mile upstream from the other two and the road which led to the barge crossing to the island and the south bank completely bypassed it. This fact was to take on significance later because there were no cases of smallpox in the north bank settlement.

I crossed the river on a small barge. The river was shallow enough for two ferrymen to push the barge across with long bamboo poles. The main part of Titilan was on the south bank, a huge sprawling village of grass huts built on top of an enormous sand dune. When I arrived on the shore, a huge crowd was waiting. The men were dressed in flowing white and indigo robes, turbans and mufflers, and the women had elaborate coiffures studded with red beads and pieces of silver.

Although the chief was the nominal head of all three settlements, it was Boubarcar Ag Yusuf, the Tuareg chief, who was very much in charge of handling the smallpox epidemic. He was a tall man in his fifties dressed in an indigo-colored turban and veil and a voluminous white robe. He had a working knowledge of French which took me by surprise.

"The French took me away from my parents when I was a child and put me in school in Bourem," he said, sensing my surprise. "We thought it was a bad thing then," he added, "but now I realize that the French were right to send me to school."

As Boubarcar was talking, I was wondering what to do first. Here I was at last. But I didn't know where to start. Then out of the corner of my eye I saw a child stick his head out of a hut's doorway. His face was speckled with numerous white dots, as if someone had splashed him with a paint brush.

"He had smallpox," said Boubarcar. "Smallpox does that to Africans. Their skin turns white for a while."

Then I remembered. "Sure," I said to myself, "vitiligo, the temporary depigmentation that occurs when the scabs fall off." I had read about it, but had never seen it before, not even in pictures.

The chief said that he had a list of everyone who had had the wind illness. His list, however, was written in Arabic along with the dates the illness started, but the dates were according to the Moslem calendar. When he told me this it gave me an idea. I would visit every hut, one by one, and look at everyone. That way I would see if it was really smallpox and chart its behavior.

I explained this to the chief and to Boubarcar and they nodded in agreement. So we started walking to the far end of the village. So did a couple of hundred other people who looked pretty healthy. They came as a chattering, swooshing entourage.

Hmm, why don't they have smallpox, I wondered. Maybe this disease isn't smallpox.

I had been taught that smallpox was a highly contagious disease. That meant it spread like wildfire. I had also been taught that it was a very lethal disease, killing almost half who got it.

I thought as I walked, if smallpox came into this village in February it should have swept through this place within two months and killed half the people.

Once in a while a child's hand touched my arm.

"They have never seen a white man before," said Boubarcar, laughing.

We arrived at the first hut. There were three little boys in it. One was covered with blisters. They were mostly on his face, arms and legs. I examined him carefully and started to run down in my mind the clinical characteristics of smallpox—"most lesions centrifugal," meaning they're on the extremities and face. "All lesions of the same age." The smallpox rash has five stages—macular, which is a flat blotch; papular, a hard bump the size of a pea; vesicular, a blister; pustular, a pus-filled blister; and finally a scab.

In chickenpox, the disease which most resembles smallpox, the lesions come out in crops, some on one day, some the next, and so on. A child with chickenpox can have papules, vesicles and scabs all at the same time. Not so with smallpox. All lesions are the same age.

"The lesions are hard," I remembered. I felt them. "Has to be smallpox. No way is this chickenpox."

But the boy's brother was covered with scabs and the other boy, also a brother, covered with areas of depigmentation.

"The anatomical distribution is classic for smallpox. But these kids got the disease at intervals of several weeks apart."

I thought hard. How could this be? If it's smallpox it's highly contagious. They should all have gotten it at the same time.

Clinically it was smallpox. But epidemiologically—that is, the way it behaved in the population—it wasn't smallpox. Boubarcar sensed my doubts.

"It is smallpox," he said. "I know, I have seen it many times before." He had the confidence of a professor on Grand Rounds in a medical center and I believed him.

I found people with smallpox in different stages of development all over the village. Some were just beginning, others were at their florid peak and others were almost over. Some cases were severe, some mild. One little girl had pocks in each eye. I knew she would recover. But she would never see again.

It's smallpox all right, I thought midway through the village. But it spreads so slowly here! You almost have to stand on your head to get it. But the crazy thing is that once you do, it can kill you.

There were 897 people in Titilan, half of them on the south bank where I started. Eighty-seven cases of smallpox occurred there and on the island.

I passed the night in one of the huts and early the next morning continued my investigation. I had to find out how many people had been previously vaccinated in their lives. I would do this by asking them and by looking for scars on their arms. I also wanted to investigate the results of Boubarcar's variolation program. This wasn't going to be easy since the commandant had threatened to fine Boubarcar if he continued variolating. And I had to get the approximate dates of onset of smallpox in each case.

I examined all of the 897 people in Titilan, and I confirmed that there weren't any cases on the north bank. I wondered to myself, why no cases there? I finally figured out the reason. Here's my report from that day:

July 21st, 1967
. . . In crossing over to the north bank, inhabitants of the south bank and island do not enter the settlement there because it is a mile north of the road and the crossing point. Also they do not get on well together and this makes for little contact. As the chief explained it, there was a big dispute over grazing rights four years ago. It was a dry year and the grass ran out on the south side of the river. The people there and the islanders wanted to graze their herds on the northern bank. This was opposed by the people of the northern settlement. Several heated palavers took place between them all. They finally came to blows. No one was killed, but the government stepped in and forced those on the northern bank to allow the others to graze their herds as they wished. The people on the northern bank had no choice but to accept. But they warned their neighbors that this defilement of their lands would anger their ancestor spirits. Since then, they have been predicting that a terrible plague will be inflicted on their neighbors by the ancestor spirits of their side of the river.

They now see the smallpox epidemic as a prophecy fulfilled because Tondibi lies on their side of the river. They claim that the Tondibi spirits have caused this epidemic on their behalf. And they are taking considerable satisfaction in the suffering of their neighbors. As they see it, they have finally been avenged. A wrong has been righted. All of this is denied by the people on the island and on the southern bank who claim that the Tondibi spirits caused this epidemic because Jeneba Maiga and her uncle defiled their sanctuary.

The credibility and esteem of the *imams* and fortune tellers on the northern bank have increased enormously since they predicted this plague. In reality, the argument which took place four years ago has

41

protected the north bank settlement from smallpox. It led to an almost complete break in social contacts with their neighbors which has made transmission of the disease to them virtually impossible.

That night I sat out in front of my hut on a straw mat and with a pen and a long yellow pad began doing some calculations. Two hundred and fifty-eight or 28.8 percent of the population had been vaccinated before, some as long as thirty years ago. Not one of these got smallpox. This was highly significant. It meant that a vaccination even decades ago gave protection here. (In India if you weren't vaccinated every two or three years you could get a bad case of the disease.) Five hundred and nineteen or 58.8 percent had never been vaccinated and sixty-five of them got smallpox and eleven died. This meant that only 12.5 percent of the unvaccinated got smallpox. The fatality rate was 16.8 percent. What all of these statistics meant was that the disease was not highly contagious, but tenacious. It spread slowly but surely, and killed occasionally. Smallpox elsewhere didn't behave like this. It spread rapidly and killed 50 percent of those who got it.

Boubarcar variolated 120 people as far as I could ascertain. All of them had had close contact with smallpox cases before their variolation. Of these 120, 18.3 percent later got smallpox, but none died. I couldn't say for sure if they developed smallpox because of being variolated or because they had had close contact with smallpox cases. I was in the same bind as those who had studied variolation in the nineteenth century! I wrote in my report:

> . . . If the figures are accepted as they are, then no great preventive advantage accrued from variolation, but among those who subsequently got the disease none died. Conversely, one cannot say that there was any great advantage from being variolated. The technique here is clean, the incisions superficial and the tissue damage small. Because the sinister implications so common in other African societies concerning variolation are absent here, one should not view it with alarm.

My last comments referred to the Shopana Cult in Dahomey (now Benin) and Nigeria. Among the Yoruba people, Shopana is the smallpox goddess whose priests cared for smallpox victims. They practiced variolation on healthy relatives of smallpox victims during rituals performed when the patient was recovering. It was also suspected, but never proven, that they saved scabs from smallpox victims. The virus survives in scabs for about six months. If patients died, the priests inherited part of their estate. So it was in their material interest to see to it that smallpox spread and that it had a significant mortality. When smallpox died out, it was suspected they started epidemics by using scabs they had saved.

Titilan was a different case altogether. Variolation was only done as a defense against an epidemic, and was otherwise never performed.

Maybe it's a different type of virus, I thought as I walked over the dunes of Titilan. It has to be different. It has to be a "zebra." I took some scab specimens from several patients, using a metal forceps, and put them in a plastic container in Titilan. Then when I got back to Bamako, I sealed them in a tin can, using a home canning kit I had brought with me. I shipped the specimens back to the laboratory at CDC in Atlanta, via the diplomatic pouch. A lot of strange things travel in diplomatic pouches, but I wondered if smallpox scabs ever had.

Three weeks later, I received a telegram from CDC saying that they had isolated smallpox virus from the scabs. Whatever fleeting doubts I may have had ever since going to Titilan were now brushed aside. But the telegram also contained some other information:

. . . virus of unusual intermediate type . . . different from variola minor, in class of its own between variola major and variola minor . . .

It *was* a "zebra"! Thinking of zebras even when dealing with a disease like smallpox had paid off in a big way. What the telegram's technical language meant was that the virus in Titilan wasn't the same type of smallpox virus found in many parts of the world. The variola major virus is the one which caused classical smallpox (until recently) throughout India and many parts of Asia. Called major, it causes serious disease and carries a very high mortality rate. At the opposite side of the spectrum is variola minor, a smallpox virus which causes a mild form of the disease. But the virus in Titilan was neither one of these two types. Its technical name is variola intermedius and it causes a midway severe form of illness. Not much was known about it at the time.

Outside of Titilan there were fifty-eight other cases, scattered up and down the river. Several cases were detected in Tondibi where Jeneba had contracted it. One of these was in a trader friend of her uncle's who frequently came to visit. The timing of his illness led me to conclude that he was in the infectious incubation period when he had contact with Jeneba. He had come to Tondibi from Tillaberi, a trading town almost three hundred miles to the south in the Niger Republic. There was a smallpox epidemic in Tillaberi at the time he was there, but it was quickly brought under control through a mass-vaccination campaign.

My job now was to get back to Bamako and send vaccinators with jet guns and vaccine to the area. By a stroke of good luck, Dr. Traore was away when I returned and with Dr. Dupont's help I was able to convince the minister to send the vaccination team out.

When the epidemic ended six weeks later, the people of Titilan and the other villages along the river thanked me. Boubarcar said it in a phrase. "You stopped what was in the wind."

But it wasn't the wind, nor spirits, nor even my search for a "zebra." It was the quick application of modern techniques and vaccine to fight a centuries-old problem in a faraway corner of the world.

CHAPTER 4

A LONG HARD ROAD

I don't remember exactly when it was that I first thought of becoming a physician, but I know I was still a child. Some of my uncles and cousins were physicians and no doubt they served, as they say today, as role models for me. What I do remember vividly is that I also always wanted to go to Africa, as far back as the first grade. It was a strange desire on the part of a six-year-old living in the borough of Queens in New York City. But not for me. My maternal grandfather was born in Algeria into a family which had spent many years in Africa. His father, who was in the French colonial service, was later killed in East Africa. My grandfather's sister, who lived with us, recounted numerous African adventure stories to me at a very early age. In all of these, my great-grandfather was heroic. And although she and my grandfather were often participating characters in these stories, they never rose to overshadow his heroic position. My great-grandfather, in another century, was either leading a military expedition against rebellious Berber nomads, defending his wife and children against wild beasts or rescuing Africans from adversity. In all these stories, he was enterprising, intelligent, highly motivated, compassionate, and . . . always successful. What a model for a young boy! I wanted to be just like him. And to be like him meant to me at that age that I had to go to Africa.

In grade school, I consumed a generous diet of books about Africa, exploration, travel and anthropology. And by the time I was midway through high school, I was quite an expert on a subject which interested few. Used-book stores were a treasure trove of old books on Africa and with my weekly allowance of a quarter I was able to buy first editions of Stanley's books and Livingstone's and those of other early explorers for less than a dollar. I used to find them at the bottom of disarrayed heaps of books in the dimly lit back aisles of stores. What excitement surged through me when I came up with a find! And for fifty cents it was mine! The book dealers were glad to be rid of these dog-eared tomes which no one else wanted. One of them used to look at me sympathetically whenever I let my fist-clenched nickels and dimes fall onto the patinated counter. "Do you really want that book?" he would ask, gently implying that no one else did. I was too shy to speak. I would nod my head up and down and then run off with my treasure.

I continued buying old books on Africa throughout the time I was in college and medical school. By then I was quite sophisticated in my knowledge of Africa and became a connoisseur in picking out books for my collection. But by 1962, when I was graduated from medical school, it was getting increasingly difficult to find old books on Africa hidden on back shelves. The "winds of change," which Harold Macmillan, the British prime minister, so aptly said were sweeping Africa, had also stirred up enormous interest in the continent. The unwanted discards I once picked up for nickels and dimes were now displayed in glass-covered bookcases, the price increased more than two hundredfold.

During my high school years I passionately wanted to be a naturalist or anthropologist of some kind working in Africa. I had become intensely interested in these two broad disciplines as an extension of my interest in Africa. But I was torn: should I become a naturalist or anthropologist, a physician or missionary? I needed help. A junior in high school, I went to see my guidance counselor, Brother Celestin George.

"I want to be a naturalist," I told him, "just like Roy Chapman Andrews."

He looked puzzled. "Who's Roy Chapman Andrews?"

I was crestfallen. How could he not know about Roy Chapman Andrews, one of my heroes?

"He's the naturalist who discovered dinosaur eggs in the Gobi Desert," I said.

"And that's what you want to do?"

"Not exactly, er, but something like that. Or, maybe do what Martin Johnson did."

His face broadened. "A wildlife photographer?"

"Well, not exactly," I said. "I really want to do something of my own, but be just like them." And with that I rested my case.

Celestin George got up from behind his desk and went over to a large dictionary, one of those *Webster's* which we put under my younger brother Gerard on Thanksgiving so he could reach the table.

"Naturalism is the belief that the natural world is the whole reality and that there is no supernatural or spiritual creation." He read it slowly with his finger moving across the page. "Have you spoken to your spiritual advisor about this?" he asked gravely and sadly.

"Er, well, no. But, Brother, I don't think naturalism has anything to do with being a naturalist."

He looked puzzled again for a moment and then went back to the dictionary and finally found the entry.

"Where did Roy Chapman train?" he asked.

"Roy Chapman Andrews," I replied, timidly correcting him.

"Whatever his name is."

"He trained at Beloit College," I said, having found that out some while back by looking Andrews up in *Who's Who.*

"How about Martin Johnson?"

"He didn't go to college. In fact he didn't even go to high school."

"Well, you had better forget about him and find out how Roy Chapman Andrews got his training."

With this brilliant recommendation I wrote to the director of admissions at Beloit College and told him that I wanted to be a naturalist just like Roy Chapman Andrews, figuring that if Roy Chapman Andrews went there and became a naturalist, so could I. The response I got back didn't meet my expectations. They offered degrees in science and the director said that they would be more than happy to set up a program for me within that broad area. But he concluded with the comment that naturalists were not created by a four-year college course but over a period of years by research and study.

Having drawn a blank I went back to Brother Celestin George for more guidance.

"No one in this school has ever wanted to be a naturalist. Why must you?"

"I just want to," I said peevishly.

"Why don't you become an engineer or go into business like most of our graduates?"

I wasn't interested in either, but didn't have the courage to tell him that. The faculty of St. Augustine's High School prided itself on a classical education and heavy concentration on mathematics. I liked Latin and English literature, but advanced calculus and trigonometry were a bore. The school wasn't equipped to permit students to select special courses. None were offered. So those of us who had interests beyond the confines of the established syllabus had to educate ourselves on our own time.

Celestin George grew exasperated. "Do your parents know about all of this?"

My parents knew all right. In fact my mother had gone so far as to say that she didn't want to see any of "those books coming into the house again." She had never been keen about my growing interest in Africa. My great-grandfather's violent death there during a native rebellion was never explained to me in detail. My great-aunt refused to talk about it, no doubt because it didn't go with her father's heroic image. My mother associated Africa with that tragedy. In retrospect I think she feared that I too would die in Africa.

Finally, Celestin George said ponderously, "Write to the American Museum of Natural History." I wrote a letter that night to the director and got a reply within a week from the head of the education department. He more or less said what the director of admissions at Beloit College told me. But I was persistent and wrote him back. This time he suggested that I come and see him.

Although I didn't realize it at the time, my meeting with Mr. Wright was a turning point. He possessed all the knowledge and qualities Brother Celestin George lacked. After we had spoken for a while, during which time he got a pretty good idea of my interests and motivation, he said, "You are someone with many interests in life. If you become a physician, you can also be an anthropologist, a naturalist, whatever else you want to be as an avocation."

No one had ever before pointed out that I might pursue several of my interests, and his words came as an exciting revelation, making me more hopeful about my future than I had ever been. None of the adults I knew had deep interests beyond the confines of their given work; and I had feared that the choice of one profession would foreclose my pursuing knowledge in another field.

"The curator of ornithology at this museum is just as much an expert on fishes as the curator of ichthyology and he in turn is a keen archaeologist."

All of this came as a great and reassuring surprise to me. Then he said something which I have never forgotten.

"Several years ago there was a man who worked here at the museum by the name of Martin Johnson."

I tingled with excitement.

"He was a wildlife photographer," Mr. Wright continued, "who had absolutely no formal training at all. He made a great contribution to natural history because he was on the scene at the right time. Almost no one has such an opportunity today. Now you have to be well trained to do the kind of field research that's needed."

I saw that while Martin Johnson's virtues could be emulated, he was no longer a viable career model, and that I would need formal training in one of my areas of interest. Mr. Wright pointed out that my inclination toward medicine was very strong and that I could easily follow such a career without giving up my other interests. My dilemma had been self-made.

When I started my undergraduate studies in the premed program at St. John's, the college was still located in a complex of old buildings in the Bedford-Stuyvesant section of Brooklyn. Ten members of my family had attended this university since the turn of the century and one had been a professor of chemistry there. The school had a fine reputation and this plus the fact that I could commute there in forty-five minutes by taking two elevated lines were the reasons I chose it. Living at home was cheaper than boarding at an out-of-town college and my family was in no position to finance my education. Although my extended family sparkled with physicians and lawyers, my father, an architect and builder, never made a comfortable living. We were always on the verge of domestic financial default. He was kind, generous, considerate and superb in his profession. But he had absolutely no business sense and always came out behind financially in his major projects.

I must have had some insight into this even when I was in high school, because I knew that if I wanted to study medicine I would have to rely on my own financial resources. All through high school, on weekends and in the summers, I worked at everything from a busboy in a Horn and Hardart Automat to messenger on Wall Street. By the time I entered St. John's I had saved up $697, which represented a lot of work considering that my take-home pay for sixteen hours on a weekend at the Automat was $13!

My first-year's tuition at St. John's was $649, which left me with some spare money for carfare. As soon as classes started I realized I had better start saving up money for the next year or there'd be none. I went into the business of cleaning and waxing cars on Saturdays at ten dollars apiece. It was rough work since the cleaners and waxes were made in paste form in those years. A lot of elbow grease had to go into this job, especially on cold winter days. One of my lawyer uncles also gave me a job on Saturdays cleaning his office, and then that first summer I worked in a commercial bank in Jamaica, Queens.

The next year summer jobs were increasingly difficult to find and the statement that landed me the bank position no longer worked. I had told them that I wanted to be a permanent employee. One of my physician uncles, "Dr. P. J.," was the medical director of Merritt, Chapman and Scott, at that time one of the largest construction and salvage companies in the country. Although his main office was in the corporate headquarters on Madison Avenue, he maintained a large clerical operation in our old family house on Sackett Street in Brooklyn.

This house had been purchased by my great-grandfather and grandfather in 1919 from the Hasbrouck family who had originally built it in 1852. It was a twenty-one-room mansion with twenty-five-foot-high ceilings. My uncle had started off his general practice there in 1921 after graduating from Cornell Medical College and later used the house for the enormous clerical operation which went along with his being in a top post in industrial medicine.

"The house has to be painted," I heard him tell my father one day. And without hesitation I said, "I can do it for you cheaper than a commercial painter."

"How much do you want?"

"Fifty-five dollars a week plus paints and all the supplies."

I then told my uncle that part of the deal had to be that I would

50

have two summers of twelve weeks each to finish the job. He agreed to this and I started painting.

By the time my senior year rolled around I had a cash surplus after paying all of my tuition and other fees. I had also gone through a lot of paint brushes. My uncle then offered me a job in the office, not painting, but examining the compensation forms which flowed in like an avalanche every day from over fifteen major projects all over the country. These projects included the Mackinac Bridge in Michigan, the Tappan Zee Bridge and the Throgs Neck Bridge in New York, the Glen Canyon Dam in Arizona and a hydroelectric dam at Lewiston, Maine.

During the years I worked in my family's old house, I developed a great attachment for it. My uncle's secretary, Suusje Karssen, and I did a great deal of research on it over the years in the archives of historical societies and even cemeteries. We discovered that the house was built by Daniel Backus Hasbrouck when he married Sarah Bergen, the daughter of Jacob Bergen, a farmer of Dutch descent who owned a huge tract of land in that part of Brooklyn. Bergen Beach and Bergen Street are named after him and his relatives. The house was built on the foundations of Jacob Bergen's farmhouse which had been constructed before the Revolutionary War. The retreating Maryland Fusiliers passed it as they fled from the advancing British and Hessians during the Battle of Long Island. There is a legend that the ghost of a Hessian soldier killed in front of the house haunts the basement.

Daniel Hasbrouck was a wealthy businessman who eventually came to own a number of surface railways in New York City. He died in the house in 1911 at the age of ninety-two. When my paternal great-grandfather and grandfather purchased the house from his daughter and grandson, they decided to preserve its interior and exterior designs. They modernized the house, with the help of my Uncle Freeman, an architect, but over the fifty-nine years it remained in my family, its basic structure wasn't altered. The house was sold by my cousins on January 6, 1978, and on that day a member of the Hasbrouck family joined me for a tour of it.

My research in a Brooklyn cemetery almost got me into serious trouble in 1977 when I was Commissioner of Health of New York City. I was tracking down the lineal descendants of Daniel Backus Hasbrouck and made arrangements with a physician friend of

51

mine, Tom Williams, to go to a Brooklyn cemetery on a Saturday afternoon. There had been a heavy snowfall a few days before so I brought a shovel along because on my previous visits I had learned that many of the grave markers are flush with the ground. I figured that I would have to do a little snow shoveling around the plot if the stone wasn't upright. This turned out to be the case.

It never occurred to us that it's pretty suspicious for someone to be seen shoveling in a cemetery on a bleak winter day. Along came a car with two security officers.

"Just what do you think you're doing there?" one of the officers shouted.

"Shoveling away snow," I replied honestly with a winded voice.

"Shoveling!" one of them exclaimed. "You can't do that. Don't you know it's against the law to tamper with a grave?"

"Tampering with a grave! Who says I'm tampering with it? I'm only clearing the snow away so I can see the marker."

I had no sooner said that then the two men go out of the car. Tom Williams, who had been near our car, started over toward me, making his way through the snow and maze of tombstones.

"You see, I'm doing research on my family house, and er, this man who is buried here, well, his grandfather built this house in 1852 on Sackett Street."

I got back a blank stare. "Research, huh?" one of them said. "That's a good one." He looked down at the ground and said, "You've been scraping a lot of earth here."

I knew now that I was in serious trouble, especially when he followed up with, "We're gonna have to take you to the front office."

I saw the newspaper headline—"Health Commissioner Accused of Grave Robbing!"

"Look, he's telling the truth," Tom Williams interjected. "Does he look like a grave robber?"

I didn't think that was an especially smart question for Tom to ask. But he didn't give them a chance to answer.

"I don't think you know who this man is," he said very proudly.

"Oh, my God!" I said to myself. "How could he be so stupid as to give away my identity?"

"This so happens to be the Commissioner of Health of New York City. Now is that the kind of person who would be grave robbing?"

52

"You're really the Commissioner of Health?" said the one who had been doing all the talking.

"Yes, I am," I replied.

"Show them your badge," Tom said, confident we had the problem licked.

"Wow, the Commissioner of Health," one of them said as they looked at my badge and ID card.

"Yeah, yeah," the other one said. "Sure that's him all right. Why, I recognize you from television. Pleased to meet you, sir," he said, shaking my hand.

"Time to skidoo," Tom whispered. And with that I excused myself and headed for the car.

In my senior year of college, I applied to six medical schools and was accepted by four. I chose to go to the State University of New York, Downstate Medical Center, in Brooklyn, New York. It had an excellent reputation and was convenient twenty-minute commute from my home. The faculty set extremely high academic standards. And the students met them, judging from their superb performance on the National Boards, examinations which medical graduates take in order to obtain licenses to practice.

During the fifth week of that first academic year a terrible tragedy struck my family. It was October 23, 1958, about nine P.M. I was studying the bones of the arm for a practical exam in Gross Anatomy the next day. My mother came into the room.

"Your father is very late tonight," she said.

"Maybe he got tied up," I said, looking at my anatomy atlas.

I heard her putting my clean shirts into the dresser drawer. "He's never this late," she said, walking slowly out of my room and down the hall.

I was worried about the Gross Anatomy exam because it was going to be tough. The way it was set up, all of the sixty cadavers in the laboratories would be exposed. Since we were being examined on the anatomy of the arm, tags would be placed on different parts of the arms of the cadavers. Next to them would be sheets with questions on them. Some would require a simple identification of the anatomical structure tagged, others would ask more complicated questions about the functions of the structure and its relationships to others.

My mother was on her way down the stairs. I could hear her feet and from the way she stepped could tell when she reached the landing which led into the dining room. The phone rang and a second later the front door bell too. My sister Joyce, nineteen, answered the phone. There was a pause. I looked up for a fraction of a second from my atlas. The silence was broken.

"Daddy's been hit by a car!"

I felt a surge of adrenalin rush through my body. I jumped up and dashed down the stairs. A policeman, who had rung the bell, was already in the living room.

"Fractured leg! Bleeding badly! Unconscious!" Joyce repeated the neighbor's report with staccato and alarm. The policeman stared at the floor. There was nothing for him to say. In the rush and confusion which followed I don't remember exactly what happened next. The policeman spoke to my mother, trying to reassure her. She leaned against one of the dining-room chairs and stared blankly ahead. He suggested that she come to the scene of the accident. She didn't reply. My youngest brother, Francis, eight, started to cry.

"You'd better come then," said the policeman to me, leading me out of the room. It was a cold autumn night and I ran into it with only a T-shirt on and an enormous sense of foreboding. The accident had happened only four blocks away from the house on a main drag known as Old South Road. My father had crossed that street for almost thirty years.

It was a chaotic scene now of blinking lights, diverted traffic and crowds of onlookers. People hovered in a large semicircle and murmured. The police captain put his arm over my shoulder when I got out of the car.

"He's going to be all right, son. Just a broken leg."

He walked me through the crowd and then I saw my father lying next to the curb. I trembled, both from the cold and the fright. He was incoherent and spattered with blood. A man put a folded blanket under his head as a pillow. His clothing had been ripped open by the impact of the car. It had struck him at full speed on the left side and hurled him thirty feet into the air. The driver was across the road, leaning against the wall of the cemetery. I heard a policeman say that he was in a state of shock. After he had struck my father, he had braked and the skid marks were visible for fifty feet. He had gotten out of his car, put his jacket over my father and run to the nearest house for help.

Until that moment I had fancied that all of my preparatory training for medicine had at least made me competent as a sort of half-baked physician. But here I was helpless, a living encyclopedia of all sorts of medical knowledge who could do no more than a well-meaning neighbor. It was a humbling experience. "All that knowledge," I said to myself, "and I can't do a damn thing!" What was the purpose of it all, organic chemistry, calculus, physics, biology? I had spent four years of my life mastering all these disciplines so that I could be a physician. And now face to face with the first real test, I couldn't use any of them to help my father.

Someone handed me what remained of my father's glasses and wristwatch. I slipped them into my pocket. "Aren't you studying to be a doctor?" he said. I nodded yes. "Maybe you can do something for him before the ambulance arrives."

It was said loud enough for everyone to hear. I crouched down next to him and took his pulse. It was all I knew how to do, an empty gesture which would do him no good, but which got me off the hook with the crowd. I felt disgusted with myself, and angry at the others.

"Here comes the ambulance!"

I looked up from my crouching position and saw it speeding down the road. The siren was blaring, but I hadn't heard it. The ambulance was a crude affair, a crumbling panel truck covered with several weeks of dust and grime. The attendant and the driver rushed out, pushing everyone aside.

"Get out of the way, kiddo," the driver shouted.

"That's his son," a policeman said.

The driver didn't reply.

The attendant was an enormous man weighing all of three hundred pounds. The driver called him Tiny. He was full of rough edges, shouting at the police and ordering the driver around with a Brooklyn accent peppered with obscenities.

"He's got a busted back. We gotta get a board under him."

Tiny told the driver to get a board from the ambulance and then he and the police hoisted my father onto it.

"My back, my back!" It was the first time my father cried out with pain.

In a matter of seconds he was carried into the back of the dilapidated ambulance. The police captain gave me a boost and Tiny pulled me in.

With the siren blaring we rushed down Old South Road to the Sunrise Highway. The ambulance rattled and jolted from the roof to the axle housings. My father's stretcher was strapped to a metal shelf attached to one wall. Anyone who wasn't strapped in would have come flying off on the first turn. I sat next to the stretcher on a metal stool which was welded to the floor. It and the shelf were the only permanent fixtures in the back of the ambulance.

This isn't an ambulance, I thought. It's a crummy junk wagon. What I did not learn until many years later was that the ambulances were supplied by the Department of Hospitals of New York City. Inspection, indeed even standards for quality, were nonexistent. In the late 1960s the Department of Hospitals was replaced by the New York City Health and Hospitals Corporation which then took over the ambulances. At the same time the Department of Health promulgated rigid standards for ambulances, effectively taking the likes of Tiny's ambulance off the road. Exactly twenty years after that ride with my father in the rickety ambulance, I became Commissioner of Health of New York City and Chairman of the Board of the New York City Health and Hospitals Corporation with sweeping powers over ambulances and their services. The ride that night which made such a terrible and vivid impression on me would deepen my determination years later to see that ambulances were equipped to help people, as the one my father rode in was not.

Tiny stood up front next to the driver, holding on to a bar attached to the roof. The window was open on his side and he shouted invectives and profanities at motorists who weren't quick enough getting out of the way.

"Get out of the way, you stupid bastard!" he blurted out just as we got to Jamaica Avenue. And then changing the tone of his voice, looked back at us and asked, "How are you doing back there?"

My father, who had suffered a cerebral concussion, became more alert. The first thing he said to me was, "I hope your mother isn't too upset by this."

Later he clutched my shirt and asked. "Am I going to die?"

He was looking straight up at me, but I couldn't bear to look at him.

"Don't be silly, you'll be all right," I said.

Deep down I wasn't sure.

The ambulance took us to a small hospital in Queens where my

Uncle Fred was an attending physician. Joyce had called him, and by the time we arrived he was at the emergency room.

The ambulance entrance was in a central courtyard stacked with garbage containers, empty tanks of bottled oxygen and some old lumber. The hospital had been enlarged several times, but all very long ago, and then renovated and rerenovated until it was a hopeless jumble of nooks and passageways. The waiting area for the emergency room was what had once been a corridor. It was a high ceiling from which old-fashioned globe lights were suspended. The paint was green, covered with a patina of grime, and the varnished woodwork was from the turn of the century. There was nothing in that setting to inspire confidence. The intern on duty, like all of the interns in this hospital, was a foreigner. He spoke with a thick Middle Eastern accent. He directed the orderly to wheel my father into a treatment room which even to my untrained eyes looked like nothing more than a first-aid station.

He told me to wait outside on one of the hard wooden benches which must have stood there for over half a century. I ignored him. Then he shouted, "Didn't I tell you to get outside!"

In retrospect, this fellow was an incompetent and had my uncle not been there things would have gone very badly. He wanted to sew up the laceration on my father's forehead even after my uncle had ascertained that my father's blood pressure was falling.

"Just put a dressing on it," I heard my uncle say. "He's in shock."

"I'm going to take him up for x-rays," the intern said.

"No, you're not," said my uncle. "We can take them later after he's stabilized. Get an intravenous into him."

There wasn't an intensive-care unit in this hospital at that time, nor in many hospitals in New York City. So my father was taken up to a medical-surgical ward where the nursing coverage was better than in other areas of the hospital. In a sense these were the forerunners of intensive care units.

Once we got up there, the intern was joined by another, this time an Italian whose English was almost as incomprehensible. He wanted a detailed history of my father's previous illnesses, something which struck me as being irrelevant to the present acute emergency. I didn't know if my father ever had chickenpox and I didn't give a damn. What bearing could that possibly have on his fractured leg and pelvis?

57

Although I could hardly think about it at the time, and was too inexperienced to recognize it, what I was witnessing was plain medical incompetence. These fellows knew medicine in theory. What they lacked was judgment. Obviously a fractured pelvis and shock take precedence over a skin laceration. That is clear to any well-trained physician. But not to these guys. Sew him up, then worry about falling blood pressure and shock!

My uncle called in two surgeons and they confirmed what he suspected. The three bones in my father's left leg were fractured, tibia, fibula and femur. In addition there were multiple fractures of the pelvis.

By three A.M., my father's condition had stabilized and it looked to me as if everything were under control. I felt reassured and decided to go home, get some sleep, take the exam and then go back to the hospital. My mother was up when I got home, but she was badly shaken. She planned to go to the hospital later in the morning. I played down the seriousness of my father's condition and I remember her saying something about getting a wheelchair for him when he came home.

It was four-thirty A.M. when I dozed off. So many thoughts were running through my head. I couldn't sleep. The events of the night seemed like some unreal happening, a nightmare which would disappear when I woke up. What will happen now, I thought. Suppose he is incapacitated? Suppose he dies? I quickly put these ideas out of my mind and tried to repeat over and over again my memorized anatomy of the arm, the origins and insertions of muscles, the nerves, the areas they stimulated, the blood vessels, the joints, ligaments and bones. But other thoughts kept crowding them out, the blinking lights, the siren, the chill wind, my helplessness, the image of my father lying in the gutter—"Am I going to die?"

The phone rang and for a fraction of time I thought my nightmare was over. The luminous dials of the clock on my dresser read five A.M. I got up and rushed down the stairs. I caught a glimpse of my sister Joyce coming out of her room. Who would be calling at this hour? Relatives would wait until after daybreak. A terrible feeling of dread came over me.

I picked up the receiver. "Hello," I mumbled softly.

"Pat, it's Uncle Fred." His voice was choked and the words came out with difficulty. Then there was a pause.

"Dad is gone."

CHAPTER 5

BECOMING A PHYSICIAN

My father's funeral took place in a torrential downpour, harsh and unrelenting. The wind swept the rain in waves across the puddle-filled streets and hammered it down on the roofs and windows of the car. How cruel, I thought, to inflict this on us too. The funeral couldn't be held in the Catholic church where my father had worshiped for thirty years because they were holding a ceremony known as Forty Hours Devotion. Church law prohibited funerals from taking place in the church at the same time. But I saw it as an antiquated practice whose result was additional hurt for the bereaved. By coincidence, John XXIII was elected Pope in Rome that very day and within a short time this practice like many others was modified.

Only in future years was I fully able to understand the magnitude of our family disaster. At the time, my feelings overpowered me. My father carried no life insurance, no pension plan, no financial equity for us to draw upon except what Social Security paid my mother and two younger brothers. The driver of the car which struck him carried the minimum level of insurance and this wasn't given to my mother until the case came up in court five years later.

We were a strongly independent family and wouldn't ask for any help. We decided to do it ourselves and we succeeded. My sister Joyce put off her desire to study nursing and went to work. Fifteen years later, and after having three children, she finally obtained her nursing degree. Some people suggested that I give up medical school and go out and get a teaching job to support the family. I gave it serious thought. But after careful analysis, I decided we could make it, even with my staying in medical school.

My mother couldn't sleep the night after the funeral; she paced up and down the hall between her room and the bathroom. About three in the morning I heard a thud. She was sprawled out on the floor unconscious. We called Uncle Fred and he came over. Her blood pressure was sky high and apparently she had suffered a stroke. She didn't wake up for almost ten hours and then in a sequel which no fiction writer would think credible it was found several weeks later that she had fractured one of her thoracic vertebrae. She was put into a brace for several months and the hypertension she never knew she had was treated.

In spite of all this I tried to hurl myself back again into the frenetic pace of medical school, where mountains of information were thrown at us every day. It wasn't easy. Contrary to rumors, the faculty of the anatomy department was understanding and arranged for me to take a make-up exam on the anatomy of the arm during the Christmas recess. But the biochemistry professor thought that my performance in the course had suffered greatly by my father's death, and no doubt it did. He gave me an unsatisfactory rating in December, when the course ended. He wasn't the cruel monster I had anticipated meeting when I went to see him about this.

"I would like you to study the material over the summer," he said. "I'm sure you can do A work."

He told me that I would have to take another final examination in September before being admitted to the second year. I did, and obtained an excellent grade.

My second year passed uneventfully. I immersed myself in the three major courses given that year, pathology, pharmacology and microbiology. And toward the end of that year, I studied physical diagnosis on the wards of the Kings County Hospital, across the street from the medical school. The course in physical diagnosis gives medical students their first contact with patients. During that course, I learned how to use the stethoscope, how to tap out the sounds of the abdomen and chest, to use the ophthalmoscope and look into patients' eyes, and to distinguish between normal body shapes and sounds and abnormal ones. The course lasted six weeks and in preparation for it we all purchased little black bags equipped with basic equipment. At last I felt like a doctor!

Like many of my classmates, I was always on the lookout for abnormal findings. I was so zealous at this that not infrequently I heard sounds which the professor said weren't there and felt lumps and bumps which turned out to be normal.

One day when we were learning to distinguish the sounds of the heart with the stethoscope, I thought I heard a diastolic murmur in the patient I was examining. Diastolic murmurs are often difficult to hear. They are sounds made by leaking heart valves. Somewhat jubilant over my discovery, I called my professor over to have him confirm it, knowing full well that he would be pleased with my diagnostic prowess at picking up a sound which is difficult to hear.

He took out his stethoscope and listened carefully to the patient's heart. He listened for almost five minutes, adjusting the instrument's ear plugs, moving the bell from one part of the chest to another and even closing his eyes so as to concentrate better. Finally he lifted his head up and said, "There's no diastolic murmur, Dr. Imperato." The patient, who had grown apprehensive throughout all of this, gave out a sigh of relief. And the professor in addressing me as "Doctor" told me that he wasn't happy over the trouble I had put him through. Whenever our professors addressed us as "Doctor" it meant that they were angry with us. It wasn't a compliment but rather a put down. Then he said to me, "Don't go looking for zebras when they're not there."

"But I was certain there was a diastolic murmur," I said.

"There isn't," he replied firmly. "Just remember that for most of your career you'll encounter common everyday problems. The unusual ones will be rare, so don't even think of them except as an afterthought." Here we were with the horses and I was seeing zebras. Maybe I was never going to be satisfied with everyday medical problems.

At the end of my second year, I applied for a summer research fellowship from the Health Research Council of the City of New York, a council I would serve on sixteen years later when I became Commissioner of Health. The fellowship carried a stipend more than enough to pay for my next year's tuition. I had arranged to carry out malaria research under the supervision of Dr. Robert Stiles, a well-known parasitologist and a professor in the medical school's Department of Microbiology and Immunology. The project I worked on tested the response of mice to malaria infections after they had been given a variety of drugs. It was an interesting experience, but I quickly learned that I preferred to work with people rather than mice.

One day during my third year of medical school, a classmate told me about a notice posted on the bulletin board. It announced overseas fellowships for medical students sponsored by the Association of American Medical Colleges and paid for by the Smith, Kline and French Laboratories. "You ought to apply for that," my classmate urged me, knowing like most of my friends of my keen interest in Africa and tropical medicine.

"Oh, I don't know," I mumbled. "I doubt I could get one."

"Why do you say that?" he asked.

"You see what it says here," I replied, pointing to a paragraph on the back page of the brochure.

"Let me see." He looked closer. "It says you have to arrange for a place to go to. Big deal. You can do that. Write to a missionary group. There's plenty of them in Africa. I know. I'm always getting letters asking for donations."

Although I was skeptical about his suggestion at the time, that night I gave it serious thought. At last I had a chance of going to Africa. It's what I had dreamed of for years. I desperately wanted to go. But I didn't know anyone in Africa. I didn't know of any medical missions whom I could ask to sponsor me. But I decided to take a bold step.

I sat down and wrote a letter to the head of the Maryknoll Fathers in Maryknoll, New York. Over the years I had seen their monthly magazine and knew that they had missions in East Africa, the part of Africa I knew best and which I so much wanted to see. But I didn't know whether or not they had medical missions there. I told him about the fellowship, a new thing at the time, and that all of my expenses would be paid for by it. All I needed was a medical mission to agree to allow me to work and study under their general supervision.

I mailed the letter the next morning and then I waited. A week went by and nothing happened. Then a few days later, a letter arrived from the administrator of the order expressing happiness with my willingness to go to Africa to study and work at one of their missions. He suggested I write to the superior of the Maryknoll Fathers in East Africa, Father Paul Bordenet, whose headquarters were in Nairobi, Kenya. I carefully composed my letter, sent it off and then waited. It was a suspenseful wait.

Within two weeks I received a letter from Father Bordenet. He said that they had a medical mission at a place called Kowak in northern Tanganyika Territory (now Tanzania). It was a remote bush post close to the Kenya border in an area which was then one of the most underdeveloped parts of East Africa.

I was full of excitement as I read the letter. I almost couldn't believe what I was reading. Father Bordenet said that they would be delighted to have me come to Kowak!

The next day I rushed into the dean's office with Father Bordenet's letter in hand and got the necessary application forms. Four pages had to be filled out, including an essay describing why I wanted to go to Africa and spend close to a year studying tropical diseases in a remote mission outpost. I could have written a book instead of a brief essay and wound up including only a fraction of my draft on the application form. There just wasn't room for the rest.

I hadn't anticipated my mother's strong negative reaction to my going to Africa. She was dead set against it. Whatever reservations she had based on family experiences were reinforced by news coverage of current events in Africa. It was 1961 and many countries had just achieved independence or were on the verge of it. The Mau Mau rebellion in Kenya was still fresh in memory; even fresher were the post-independence massacres in the Congo. It was my bad luck that a television program on Africa was aired two days before I was due to send in my application forms, concentrating on the terrible Congo massacres as well as the condition of workers in South African diamond mines. My mother sat glued to the television. The story that unfolded wasn't reassuring. Even I had trepidations.

But a detailed letter from Father Bordenet stressing that Kowak was in a quiet corner of Africa set me back on course. It was so peaceful there he said that I would be able to see zebras grazing on the plains below Kowak late in the afternoon. I thought it funny that he mentioned zebras. If I won the fellowship, I would be heading for a part of the world full of zebras of all kinds. I would see them, hear them and have to think about them. The rare and unusual in the United States would be common there. I had to prepare myself for a complete change of outlook.

I submitted my papers to the dean's office and then waited. A month went by and then two. As the weeks passed I tried not to think about the fellowship, to prepare myself for an unfavorable ruling by the selection committee. But I couldn't shed my strong feelings of excitement about going to Africa. So the device just didn't work.

Then one day on into the third month, the dean's secretary came into the cafeteria late in the afternoon. I was sitting at a table with some of my classmates discussing our course in psychiatry. There was excitement in her steps as she walked toward the table.

"Have you heard the news?" she said with a broad smile. "No." I smiled back, knowing simultaneously what the news must be.

"You've been awarded the Smith, Kline and French Fellowship."

"Really?"

"Yes," she replied reassuringly. "We just received the letter."

I was overjoyed! At last I would go to Africa!

I became a celebrity in the medical school overnight. No one had ever gone to Africa, not even faculty members. This was the era before the Peace Corps and widespread tourist travel to Africa. By any stretch of the imagination, it was an unusual event. A press release from the medical school ushered in feature stories in all the major New York City newspapers. Today they would hardly take notice of some med student going to Africa!

I sat through the remaining weeks of school thinking of Africa. Hundreds of images flashed through my mind, images from the books I had purchased as a boy, from the movies I had seen in high school and from the stories my great-aunt had told me long ago. With each passing day my excitement intensified. It was an excitement of a nature I've never experienced again, full of anticipation and at the same time satisfaction. I was on the threshold of a thrilling adventure. It was my boyhood dream and I had made it come true.

It took a long time to get from New York to Nairobi in 1961. I flew out of Idlewild Airport to Rome via Paris on a Boeing 707 and then from Rome to Nairobi on a DC-6 via Cairo and Khartoum. The Rome-Nairobi stretch took twenty hours. I had never flown before in my life, so what may have been a tedious trip to many was an adventure for me. Early in the morning the plane flew past the snow-capped peak of Mount Kenya and then glided down into Embakasi Airport at Nairobi. What a thrill it was for me, twenty-four years old, to set foot in East Africa!

My feelings were very different in 1977, when as Commissioner of Health of New York City and a married man of forty-one, I returned to Nairobi after an absence of sixteen years. Then I saw Kenya through the eyes of someone who had lived in Africa for six years. Nothing startled me. I was accustomed to the unusual, to the exotic. But my wife, who had never been to East Africa, now experienced the same feeling of thrill I had had in 1961.

"Father Bordenet is down in Tanganyika," said Brother Ronald, who came out to the airport to meet me. "But I'll get you all set for your trip there." And some trip it was to be, five days by train, boat and jeep. I wrote the following description of this proposed journey in my book *Bwana Doctor:*

> . . . It requires about five days of travel by train, lake steamer and jeep to reach the interior of Tanganyika Territory, where the Kowak Mission is located. . . . I had planned to travel the 300 miles to the port of Kisumu on Lake Victoria via the old Uganda Railway. At Kisumu I would board the sixty-year-old German steamer *Usoga,* which would then carry me down into Tanganyika Territory, to a small port called Musoma. A day's trek through the bush by jeep would bring me to my ultimate destination, the Kowak Mission.

Kowak was certainly a far-off corner of the world, in the middle of nowhere, right on the edge of the now famous Serengeti Plains, known for their abundant wildlife. The Kenya border was but a few miles away and I crossed over it through the bush numerous times during the course of my medical work. Disease does not respect boundaries.

Unlike anything I was to see later in West Africa, this mission wasn't in a town or a village. It was just there all by itself, serving a sparse population of Luo farmers who lived close to the shores of the lake and Bakuria herdsmen who lived on the plains. In retrospect, living conditions were very tough. The religious Fathers and Sisters there used kerosene lamps, washed their clothing in the river and drank rainwater which they collected in large cement cisterns placed at the corners of the tin-roofed buildings. The runoff during the rainy season had to carry them through the long dry season.

The year which I spent in East Africa taught me more about disease and suffering in the tropics than I could ever have learned from reading textbooks and journals dealing with tropical diseases. Life wasn't separated into a world of yesterdays, todays and tomorrows, but into a repetitive pattern of todays where the struggle for survival took precedence over everything else. Children died easily here and few adults lived to old age. Ancient beliefs in gods and spirits were strong. People said they lived in the sky and traveled on the wind. I quickly learned that I had better understand these beliefs and how they influenced people's attitudes toward illness and its treatment and how they determined the African's perception of Western medicine.

I lacked the training and experience to fully study and interpret these beliefs. But as an amateur anthropologist I had a fairly open mind about them and was willing to learn whatever I could. At first I was baffled that people didn't see the logical connection between disease and its causation and between treatment and cure. But after a while I learned that these connections weren't logical in an African context, in a world where disease was due to supernatural causes. I wrote the following in my diary:

August 26th, 1961
. . . By a peculiar set of circumstances, the coming of modern medicine to Kowak has enhanced the reputations of various witch doctors. Impatient for a rapid cure, many of the infectious disease patients leave the dispensary before our antibiotic therapy has taken effect. They go to witch doctors, follow their instructions in performing various rituals, and then when our drugs are making known their curative effects, conclude that the witch doctor has cured them. . . . To make matters worse, many of the natives then return to tell us that our medicines are no good and that they've been cured by witch doctors.

Sister Mary Reese, a woman with excellent training and vast experience as a nurse, ran the dispensary and small hospital with the assistance of three other sisters and an African staff. We treated around a hundred people a day at the dispensary. I realized through treating them the magnitude of suffering in this part of the world. It was staggering! Each morning, within a three-hour period, I treated people with leprosy, malaria, intestinal worm infections, dysentery, encephalitis and many other tropical diseases. And during the afternoons, I worked with Mary Reese and the other sisters caring for the patients who had been admitted to the small hospital. The women were housed in a large tin-roofed building which contained twenty beds. The men stayed in a large round straw-roofed hut which had room for six mats. A far cry from Kings County Hospital!

I knew that much could be done to thwart disease in this part of the world, but to be effective, one had to be well trained, skilled, dedicated and understanding of the beliefs and attitudes of the people one would be serving. As I worked with Mary Reese and the sisters, I recognized that I wasn't skilled enough yet. That would come with training and experience, I knew. Time and again I saw that good intentions weren't enough in the remote bush. In the future I would have to go armed with all the assets I could muster.

This was brought home to me one July afternoon as I was driving back to Kowak from the Kenya border area. I had just crossed the Munagusi River, and with the Land-Rover in first gear, was struggling to get up the steep embankment. A crowd of people were at the top, making frantic motions for me to stop. They told me there was a woman nearby who had been in labor for several days. "But the baby won't come out," one of them added.

"Where is she now?" I asked.

An old woman pointed to a heavy growth of thorn bush two hundred yards away. When I reached the area I found the woman lying on the bare ground in a state of complete exhaustion. Nearby was a local "ambulance," two parallel bicycles with sisal poles rigged between them. It was an ingenious invention on which patients were often brought to us at Kowak.

Apparently the woman's family had started off with her early in the morning and had covered close to six miles at the point I met them. There were still ten miles left to Kowak.

"We thought we would try again to get the baby out," said the old woman. She said that they had been pounding on her abdomen with their fists. In fact, during the previous two days, they had been standing on her abdomen and attempting to push the baby out by digging their heels into the area around the top of the uterus.

"We don't have to go to Kowak now," said the old woman to me. "You are a *bwana m'ganga* [doctor] and you can pull the baby out right here."

What! I thought. She has to be out of her mind.

She wasn't. To her way of thinking I could do anything because I was a doctor.

"I'll have to take her to Kowak," I told the woman's family. They were disappointed because they thought I could deliver the baby right there and save them all a trip. I had them place the woman in the back of the Land-Rover and then we set off for Kowak. The old woman rode on the front seat with me and my interpreter. She said that the woman had been in labor for about a week. She had had eight previous babies, all of whom were delivered without any problem. I was puzzled by this. Why should she be having trouble delivering this baby, I wondered.

When I got back to Kowak, Mary Reese was away in a nearby village. I examined the woman in the small delivery room of the hospital and found that the baby's head was well engaged in the pelvis. So it's not a breech," I said to myself, for that's what I had thought. The fetal heartbeat was miraculously strong. I didn't know what to do next.

In a couple of hours the rest of the woman's family arrived. They were surprised that I hadn't delivered the baby yet. "Why can't you just reach up there and pull the baby out?" the old woman said. "You are a *bwana m'ganga*," she added, implying I wasn't living up to my position.

When Mary Reese arrived she confirmed my findings. "The baby's head is probably just a little too big," she said, taking off her gloves.

"That can't be," I replied. "She's had eight previous children and never had any trouble."

Mary Reese smiled. "I'll bet you the head is just a little bit too big. Her other babies may have been much smaller and that's why they made it through the pelvis."

I didn't agree with her. It had to be something else—like poor labor.

There were no operating facilities at Kowak and the only way of

68

saving the baby and the mother was through a Caesarean section. She had to be taken to the Mennonite Hospital at Shirati, where a surgeon was in residence. Shirati was a full day's trip from Kowak, a treacherous trek criss-crossed by several large rivers. We started off the next morning at sunrise.

By noon the woman was operated on and delivered of a big ten-pound baby who had a pretty big head. "You see," Mary Reese said, "I told you the head was too big."

There was a virtual epidemic of tetanus around Kowak that summer, among children who had been recently circumcised. The Bakuria and Basembeti people who lived in the region circumcised boys and excised girls when they reached puberty. The male circumcisions were performed with knives, the boys standing during the procedure. The female excisions, however, were done with razor blades. Knives were used previously, but the women who did the operation told me that razor blades were easier to use in cutting off the clitoris. In both boys and girls, the surgery was crude and septic. We spent a lot of time treating the complications—wound infections, hemorrhage and tetanus. Most of the children who developed tetanus died.

The surgery was part of a far greater social event, the entry of youngsters into the world of adults. As an amateur anthropologist I was keenly interested in the customs associated with this ceremony and had respect for them. But as a physician in training, I also had to deal with the serious medical complications of circumcision. The end result was that I had very mixed feelings about the continuance of the practice.

Christian missionaries in this border country between Kenya and Tanganyika were strongly opposed to circumcision and excision. But many Christian children had to undergo the operations because of public-opinion pressure from the non-Christian majority and because no one could marry until they had been circumcised or excised. This brought the missionaries of all denominations into sharp conflict with the tribal elders. Government officials, while sympathizing with the missionaries, adopted a hands-off policy. But the future government of independent Tanzania later took strong measures to curtail the practice. What I didn't know at the time was that I was witnessing ceremonies which would soon become historical. I recorded the following in my diary:

* * *

69

August 15th, 1961

. . . Trekked to the village of the female circumciser before dawn and met up with a hyena down in a gully. The village was surrounded by a wall of candelabra cactus almost twenty feet tall. It took a while to gain entry because the main gate was blocked with numerous logs. Once I got inside I found the place bustling with activity. Sixteen girls were going to be excised. They had spent the night in a cold stream so as to anesthetize themselves and make their tissues soft and easy to cut. The girls looked terribly frightened.

A group of old women went into a hut on the other side of the square and then the female circumciser invited me in. The old women had arranged themselves in a semi-circle in the center of the hut. The female circumciser sat down in front of them with her back to them. In a couple of minutes an old woman crawled toward the door and called for the first girl to be brought in. She came with a female relative to support her. The missionaries call these women "circumcision mothers," making them akin to god mothers, since they and the girls have a special social relationship for the rest of their lives.

The girl was put into a semi-reclining position, leaning back against her "circumcision mother" who supported her from a kneeling position. The girl's wraparound was removed. The circumciser spread the girl's legs and opened her vulva with her left hand, groping for the clitoris. I don't know how she could see what she was doing. It was so dark in the hut and the air was full of smoke from the old women's pipes. They strained their necks to look both at what was going to happen and at the girl's face. Any girl who cries out is subject to ridicule later in life and the derisive remark: "She cried at her circumcision."

The girl dug her fingers into the earthen floor as she was cut, jerked a little and grimaced, but didn't cry out. Still bleeding she was then taken outside.

The girls who were Christians went home immediately, whereas those who weren't remained in the female circumciser's village for a couple of weeks performing a number of rituals and receiving instruction about their future roles as women, wives and mothers. In both groups, the operation site was inspected by the old women of the family to make sure that all of the clitoris had been removed. Not infrequently, girls were sent back to the circumciser for a second operation when the old women thought that more could be cut off. This often resulted in removal of the upper portion of the wall of the vagina and damage to the opening of the urethra.

70

The wounds were routinely treated with herbs and cow dung, which resulted in terrible infections. The septic nature of the operations and the extensive tissue damage also created the right conditions for the tetanus organism to grow. Sometimes large arteries and veins were cut and children bled to death. This was more common among girls than boys, since the external female genitals have an extensive blood supply. It was impossible to accurately estimate the complication rate, but I was able to ascertain that close to 5 percent of the Christian children died.

Once they recovered from the operation, the children decorated their bodies with white kaolin and red ocher and dressed in colorful cowhide skirts, beads and feathers. The boys carried bows and arrows and tried to kill birds and small animals to demonstrate their prowess. These children traveled in large groups, going from village to village, soliciting gifts. I would often come across them in the bush. They were quite an impressive sight, one which would have pleased any anthropologist doing research. But I saw the other side of this scene as well and it wasn't pretty.

Father Bordenet had wisely failed to mention that hyenas howled beneath the windows at Kowak at night and that leopards prowled the grounds. There were many snakes in the area as well, especially puff adders. Puff adders have a habit of lying on paths at night and most patients I treated were bitten because they accidentally stepped on them. People believed that the fangs remained in the wound and would demand that I take them out! One of the sisters at the dispensary faced this problem so often that she finally devised an ingenious solution. She got a pair of snake fangs, put them in a bottle and then produced the bottle every time a patient asked to see the fangs that she had taken out.

There was a great expanse of uninhabited country to the east of Kowak. It was a high dry land of tall grass and great umbrella trees, of cool breezes and deep blue skies. Beyond it lay the Serengeti Plains and to the north the broad valley of the Mara River. It was the home of antelope, giraffe, gazelle and elephant. Zebra, lion and rhino and all the other animals lived undisturbed by man in this parcel of earth set apart by river and swamp, mountains and time. For me it was the Africa of yesterday, the high pristine plateau, where man was but an occasional visitor and had no long-lasting effect on a cycle in which nature turned over on itself.

71

It was into this beautiful Africa that I went one day to take pictures of wildlife. I went in by way of Iramba, and drove across the trackless grasslands where the scent of wilderness was in the air. The horizons were dotted with herds of topi antelope and umbrella-shaped mimosa trees whose broad shadows stretched across the yellow grass and gave shelter to clusters of zebra and gazelle. There was something eternal about this place, about the sounds which danced across the grass, its sheer expanse and throbbing life. There was no sense of human warmth and yet there was a feeling of overpowering awe.

This was the Africa which Martin and Osa Johnson and many others saw. They tried to capture it on film, describe it with words, bring it to others to share and enjoy. But it had to be experienced, heard and smelled. It was as much the air and the sky and the sounds of life as the visual image of herds of gazelle. I had never had such an experience before. Man was of no importance here. He was but an intruder who if removed would not be missed.

I went into this country with Kambaragi, a Bangirimi guide, who was then an old man with three wives. I wasn't much interested in hunting, but I took along a 375 Magnum which belonged to Bill Tolbert who was in charge of the mission at Iramba. It was a large bore gun, used for hunting elephant. The thinking was that if it could kill elephant, it could kill anything else. But I found this rifle hard to use because it was almost as tall as I was.

We headed north, close to the Kenya border, toward the area which would in later years be designated as the Masai-Mara Game Park. Kambaragi's ear lobes had been stretched when he was a youth. He told me that the right one had been slit in half a few months before. He didn't bother to go on and explain as Bill Tolbert later did that an enraged husband did it because Kambaragi was fooling around with his wife. It was a great disgrace among the Bangirimi to have a broken ear lobe. Kambaragi had taped the two loose ends together, but they kept coming apart. As we drove along, he asked me if I could sew the loose ends together. Looking back, I probably could have, given a decent operating room. But out there in the wilderness, it was out of the question. A day didn't go by though that Kambaragi didn't raise the issue time and again. I had to admire his tenacity.

We made our camp inside a thicket, next to a waterhole, which

Kambaragi said was the safest place around. Safe from what, I wondered. Kambaragi was benign and vague in his response. But when he said there weren't any lions in the area or leopards, I had reason to doubt him since earlier in the day we almost collided with a herd of buffalo emerging from some thick bush. Kambaragi had told me only hours before that there were no buffalo in the area! This camp didn't have the comforts of those set up by Nairobi-based safari outfitters. But what it lacked in comforts was more than compensated for by Kambaragi's ingenuity.

He made a table by placing four forked stakes in the ground, crossing each pair with a small branch on top of which he laid two planks brought out from the mission. My tent consisted of an old tarpaulin draped over a branch and staked into the ground. Kambaragi built a fire, set up my cot under the tarp and then heated up some canned goods. As darkness fell, I began to feel apprehensive. There was no moon that night, and the air was full of noises, some familiar and many strange. I scanned the light of my flashlight beam outside the thicket and picked up pairs of shining eyes. Kambaragi said they were hyenas and jackals, nothing to worry about since he would keep the fire going all night. I asked him again about lions. It seemed to me that I was a perfect dish, sleeping up on a cot under a scanty tarp. Kambaragi said there were no lions. But he suggested that I place the rifle standing up next to my cot. In case there were any and they came along, seeing the rifle, they would leave! At least this was Kambaragi's logic.

I had never heard a real lion roar, not even in a zoo. But shortly after midnight, I woke up because of a loud, repetitive grunting sound. Kambaragi was fast asleep and the fire was down to some warm embers. I shook the old man, but by the time he was fully awake the sound stopped. I didn't get very much sleep after that, even though the fire was rebuilt. I heard the sound again and so did Kambaragi. He told me to go back to sleep, that the sound was from a herd of wildebeest nearby. Looking back over subsequent years of African experience, I am convinced that it was a lion grunting some miles away. In 1977, when I was with my wife in the Meru Game Park in central Kenya, we heard the same kind of grunting and again when we were at the base of Mount Kilimanjaro. In both instances it was a lion. But we were safely sitting in the lounge of a safari lodge. The old man didn't want to frighten me, I think, seeing how anxious I was. And he knew from the loudness of the sound that the lion was some distance away and unlikely to come near. I lay awake most of the night, longing for my bed at Kowak where at least the hyenas were outside a window I could close.

The next morning we started off across the plains to take pictures. In addition to wanting me to fix his ear, Kambaragi now said he wanted my pith helmet. No way was I going to give it up. I had gone through a lot of trouble to get this one because they were extremely scarce then. Europeans simply didn't wear them anymore because ordinary lightweight hats were more effective against the sun and more comfortable. But I was oblivious to this and felt that I had to wear one since I was in Africa. I was living my boyhood dreams to the fullest! What a silly sight I must have been, walking around in that pith helmet! After a lot of effort, a friend of Mary Reese had found this hat in Mwanza, a town at the southern shore of Lake Victoria. It made its way to me over a period of a month, relayed north by traveling groups of missionaries. I was so overjoyed when I got it that it became a permanent part of my anatomy.

"No wonder your face is half hidden in the photographs!" my wife said, laughing, years later in our Manhattan apartment. I had found my pith helmet in a closet and put it on for her. "It's a full size too big!" she said.

Kambaragi grudgingly settled for a golfer's hat which I carried along as a spare. What a sight he was, stalking animals on the green grass of Africa!

Taking pictures was all well and good, but Kambaragi wanted to know why I hadn't shot anything. I wasn't especially interested in hunting and in fact in later years became very active in many wildlife conservation efforts. But this was a different era, when Africa's wildlife still seemed limitless to the naive.

I finally decided that I would have to shoot something, preferably a zebra, since there were so many of them and I thought they would be an easy target. We drove north across the plains and within a few minutes spotted a herd of about thirty. Kambaragi and I started stalking them through the thick bush. It was difficult to get close to any species in this wilderness. They were unfamiliar with man and would run off as soon as one got within a few hundred yards of them. How surprised I was in later years when I rode through the game parks in Kenya and came to within a few feet of most animals.

It was midday and the heat waves were strong. Through the telescopic sight of the rifle, the zebra looked like they were jitterbugging. How can I take aim, I kept thinking. The heat waves are too strong.

"Piga, Piga!" Kambaragi said in Swahili, urging me to shoot. I couldn't bring myself to pull the trigger. The zebra ran off. Kambaragi shook his head in disgust as we walked back to the truck and kept muttering that I wasn't a big *bwana*. How could he hold his head erect among his friends if his *bwana* couldn't even shoot a zebra? Kambaragi lived in a world where a man wasn't a man if he didn't know how to hunt. I knew I would have to prove my prowess in order to preserve my social status.

So the next day I gave it another try. We tracked down a herd of zebra by using the truck, then got out and stalked them for almost a half hour. We got very close to them because we were downwind and they didn't sense our presence. By this time I was tired and wanted to rest. It was hot and the tsetse flies were a nuisance. Kambaragi told me to take aim. I decided to place the barrel of the gun in the crotch of a tree. It was heavy and I needed some support in order to take steady aim. A lot of good I would have been if a rhino or a lion were charging us!

"Piga, Piga!" Kambaragi whispered, putting his fingers in his ears to deaden the blast from the rifle. I took aim at a big chunky zebra. Even so, he was dancing up and down in the heat waves which lay between him and my gun sight. It was a perfect shot and I was confident I wouldn't miss. I pulled the trigger and heard the boom and felt the recoil.

"Mzuri sana, sana—very, very good," Kambaragi said happily, clapping his hands. The herd ran off, leaving the wounded animal behind. We got into the truck and drove toward it. As we approached, I realized that this wasn't the animal I had aimed at. Kambaragi shook his head with good reason.

"Toto punda milia—a baby zebra," he moaned in Swahili. It wasn't exactly a baby, more of an adolescent. But people like Kambaragi didn't make such fine distinctions. The poor animal just stood there a few hundred yards away, staring at us, a big wound in its belly. I felt pretty rotten.

The zebra galloped off and Kambaragi and I followed it on foot for close to a quarter of a mile. Finally, fatigued from internal bleeding, the zebra stopped. There weren't any trees around with a crotch where I could place the rifle, so I decided to sit down on the ground and take aim. I really felt awful about the zebra. But now I had no choice. I fired at the chest, but instead the bullet hit the animal on the back. The zebra fell to the ground. Kambaragi rushed up and cut the struggling zebra's throat, something which took me by surprise because this is a Moslem practice and Kambaragi was a Christian, or so he said.

"It is not so easy to catch zebra," Kambaragi said laughingly. He was right, not only about the live zebras on the plains of Africa, but as I thought in later years, about medical zebras which elude most modern physicians.

CHAPTER 6

PUBLIC HEALTH AND DISEASE DETECTION

I returned to the United States after a year in Africa feeling un-fulfilled. But I knew that I would have to continue my training if I were to go back to Africa in the future and do something meaning-ful.

Tropical medicine isn't one of those medical specialities for which there is a standardized training track. And by the time I started my internship, it had really become more of a curiosity for American physicians than a viable field in which to make a living. Complicating matters, "tropical medicine" brings together many different types of scientists—physicians, parasitologists, virolo-gists, bacteriologists and others. Physicians, in fact, form only a small segment of those who consider tropical medicine an area of major interest. The field in the United States has been historically dominated not by doctors but scientists whose chief interests are in laboratory research. While this research deals with the prevailing diseases of the tropics, it has usually been far removed from any-thing that could have practical application for suffering people. Those like myself interested in treating these diseases or in pre-venting them found little to inspire them in the bulk of the Ameri-can research publications devoted to tropical medicine.

I was also interested in internal medicine, a sort of natural com-

77

bination since, as I'd learned in Africa, internal medicine in the tropics *is* tropical medicine! People often ask me "What is internal medicine?" It is not such an easy question to answer in layman's terms. Basically internists are to the adult population what pediatricians are to children. They have received several years of training after their internship, which gives them skills and knowledge generally above that of the old-time general practitioner. In recent years, internists have increasingly become the family doctor and personal physician, replacing the general practitioners who have gradually disappeared. Some internists go on for additional training in what is called a subspecialty such as gastroenterology, allergy, infectious diseases, hematology and so forth. To be a good internist, a doctor must master an enormous body of facts, possess keen diagnostic skills and be a warm, caring human being.

I decided to do my internship at the Long Island College Hospital in Brooklyn, one of the main teaching hospitals of the Downstate Medical Center, with an excellent staff of attending physicians and a fine reputation. Having great appeal for me was the fact that within its department of internal medicine was a tropical-disease section which operated one of the few tropical-disease clinics in New York City. Most of the patients were either seamen who came from the nearby waterfront or recent immigrants from Puerto Rico who lived in the surrounding neighborhood.

I realized then that while one could acquire the knowledge, judgment and ability to be a tropical-disease specialist in the United States, one couldn't do much with it here. There simply weren't enough people sick with the so-called tropical diseases. A doctor's dilemma!

My experience in East Africa taught me that to be good in tropical medicine, one had to first become a specialist in internal medicine and practice tropical medicine as a subspecialty. And to practice it in a meaningful way, I knew that I couldn't do it on Park Avenue, but only in Africa where there was a crying need for someone with those abilities.

So after finishing my internship, I did two-years' residency training in general internal medicine at Long Island College Hospital. I had decided during my internship that I would round out my training with a year of study in tropical medicine. This way I would fulfill all of the requirements of the American Board of Internal

Medicine and at the same time develop my knowledge in the subspecialty of my choice.

There was only one university in the United States which gave a degree in tropical medicine: Tulane in New Orleans. At that time the program was administered by the Division of Hygiene and Tropical Medicine which later became the School of Public Health and Tropical Medicine. Only physicians were eligible for the year of training at the end of which they were given the degree of Master of Public Health and Tropical Medicine.

I was scheduled to finish my two-year residency in internal medicine at the Long Island College Hospital in June of 1965. In late 1964, I filled out the application forms for the program at Tulane and then started looking for a way of financing this year of study.

"We've never had an applicant who wanted to study tropical medicine," said the elderly physician in a blue pin-striped suit.

I responded with a nervous smile.

"We just interviewed an applicant," said another member of the committee candidly, "who wants to do DNA research in England."

"Most of our applicants are of that type, you know," added the elderly physician in the blue pin-striped suit.

"Where did you go to college?"

"St. John's."

My questioner smiled. "That's a wonderful school. Almost ivy league, I'd say," and leaning toward the chubby physician next to him, said, "wouldn't you say so, Carl?"

"Why, yes, it's a magnificent school."

It didn't take a genius to figure out that they were thinking of another St. John's. Not the one I went to.

"How far is it from Baltimore?"

"Baltimore?"

An embarrassed hush fell over the conference table.

"It's in Brooklyn and Queens."

"Well, now," said the chairman, clearing his throat and the awkward atmosphere as well, "let's talk about your plans to study tropical medicine."

His name was Dr. Milton Raisbeck, and he was an eminent New York cardiologist, partial sponsor of the Glorney-Raisbeck Fellowship of the New York Academy of Medicine. The fellowship gave a grant of $7,500 for a year's study or research in the general area of medicine. This was a generous sum since residents in internal medicine like me were earning about $3,000 a year at the time.

I had applied for this fellowship, not especially optimistically. The competition was tough and while waiting outside the oak-paneled conference room I met some of the other candidates. One was from the Rockefeller Institute, another from Columbia University and a third from the Sloan-Kettering Institute. I felt outdistanced.

It was a long subway ride home on the IRT Lexington Avenue line, down the length of Manhattan to the Wall Street area where I changed for the Independent line which took me out to southern Queens via Brooklyn: an hour and fifteen minutes.

"How was it?" my mother asked as I put my coat in the hall closet.

I shrugged. Before I could say more than a discouraged "Okay," the phone rang and I picked it up lethargically.

"Dr. Imperato, please." I didn't recognize the voice.

"Speaking."

"This is Dr. Raisbeck from the New York Academy of Medicine."

I checked to see if my wallet was in my pocket. Maybe it had fallen out on the chair during the interview or maybe I had lost something else.

"In my specialty," he went on to say with determination in his voice," I am accustomed to giving people bad news."

Thoughts whizzed through my mind. How cruel. A letter saying no would have done.

"So you can imagine what a pleasure it is for me to give someone good news."

I was overcome and didn't exactly hear the rest of what he said, but it was something like, "You've been awarded the Glorney-Raisbeck Fellowship for 1965–66. Will you accept?"

"Accept, well, of course, accept. Yes, I'll accept."

I couldn't believe it. I was awarded the fellowship. Now I could afford to go to Tulane. It was the first really nice thing that had happened in my life in a long time. I jumped into the air and gave out a yell when I put the phone down. For years my mother would say,

"I never saw him so happy as when he was awarded that fellowship."

The academic year at Tulane began in September, but I had arranged with the dean, Dr. C. S. Miller, to begin July 1. Dr. Miller was British and had spent many years in India. He candidly told me over the phone that contrary to popular belief among physicians, there was little tropical disease to be seen in New Orleans.

"There is probably much more there in New York," he added, "but not really enough to train you well. You really have to spend time in the developing world, under good supervision and in a good center. So I suggest we send you to Cali, Colombia, for two months or so."

Although I didn't know it at the time, Tulane operated an International Center for Medical Research and Training in Cali in conjunction with the Universidad del Valle, which had a very good hospital.

"But I don't speak Spanish!"

"You must speak Italian with a name like Imperato."

"I don't."

"Not a word?"

"Not a word. But," I added, "I'm fluent in French."

"Well, no matter, you'll make out well enough with your French."

The closest I had ever gotten to South America was traveling for a few days in 1964 and 1965 to the Caribbean on the Los Angeles Dodgers' plane. As a medical resident I got a month's vacation each year and during that time worked as the camp physician in Dodgertown, the team's training center in Vero Beach, Florida. I had been selected for the job by Dr. Herbert Fett, who was then the chief of orthopedic surgery at Long Island College Hospital and the team's former physician when they were in Brooklyn. Each year he recommended a physician to Walter O'Malley, the team's owner.

Walter O'Malley and his son Peter often traveled to Africa on big-game hunting trips and this gave us a common interest. In addition to that, Walter O'Malley was keenly interested in medicine and so over the years our friendship grew. During spring training he would take me with him on the Dodger plane, *Kay O,* whenever

81

he flew down to the Caribbean and there I was given a few days to look into local medical problems and practices which certainly broadened my knowledge.

As it turned out, my experience at the university hospital in Cali was an excellent one. I teamed up with two Colombian physicians who spoke good English and because of them was able to participate in rounds, conferences and clinic sessions. I saw patients with most of the major tropical diseases, learned their diagnosis and treatment through firsthand empirical experience and came to realize as I had never before that the conquest of these diseases lay not in treating them but in preventing them.

At Tulane we were taught management, law, economics, systems analysis and decision-making techniques, geared at training us to be first-rate administrators. But throughout all of this, compassion and the individual patient were never forgotten. As public-health specialists we would be making decisions which would affect the lives of large numbers of people whereas the average medical practitioner has impact on the lives of only a few thousand people during a career several decades long. Moreover, the private practitioner treats illness once it has occurred in an individual patient, but the public-health specialist's orientation is to prevent disease in masses of people. Both are needed.

In biostatistics, I learned basic principles, how to construct graphs and charts, tabulate data, analyze them and test them for significance. But more importantly I learned how to use biostatistics to measure the health of masses of people. Data flow into health departments and into Washington, D.C., daily. Public-health specialists know how to examine them, decipher their messages and draw conclusions from them, much the same way the practicing physician deciphers the signs and symptoms of an individual patient.

Epidemiology had always been a sort of abstraction for me, a dusty concept hastily mentioned in half a breath in medical school. I knew that epidemiologists investigated epidemics and controlled them and that they were known as medical detectives. But until that time I had never met a real, live epidemiologist nor seen one at work. I had seen surgeons operate, pediatricians treat children for infections of different kinds and internists care for the victims of

82

heart attacks and strokes. But I had never seen anyone investigate and control an epidemic. My insularity wasn't unique. Few practicing doctors have any direct contact with epidemiologists, since few are ever involved in a meaningful way with the investigation and control of outbreaks and epidemics.

When I was a medical student it was explained that epidemiology is the science of epidemics. More broadly defined, it is the science which concerns itself with the natural history of disease as it is expressed in groups of people related by common factors of age, sex, race, location or occupation as distinct from development of disease in the individual. As a medical student I found little in all of this to which I could relate and certainly no inspiration to become an epidemiologist.

I learned at Tulane that while epidemiology is a profession for some, occupying all of their working hours, for others it is a skill which is used as needed. No wonder there is much confusion about the nature of epidemiology. Some of the leading epidemiologists in the United States are also pediatricians or internists. Others, such as the epidemiologists of the Center for Disease Control in Atlanta, Georgia, restrict themselves to epidemiology.

The key to being a crackerjack medical detective is in knowing your facts and having an inquisitive mind. Those who have the former and not the latter are washouts. No lead, however small, must ever be viewed as insignificant. And very often a complex chain of events and confluence of unimaginable circumstances result in epidemics.

"Shoe-leather epidemiology, ladies and gentlemen, is how you do it." It was with these words that our professor described the process of walking, snooping, opening closets and garbage cans, asking the improbable because the improbable is what usually takes place and making a pest of ourselves to everyone until we found clues which made sense. It means going down a lot of blind alleys, on a lot of wild-goose chases, of appearing to be a fool and of putting oneself in uncomfortable situations. It means thinking of zebras when others think of horses and often being alone in doing so.

By the time spring rolled around I decided to join either the Army or the United States Public Health Service. It was the height of the Vietnam War and physicians were being drafted into military service for two years. It was just a matter of time before I would be drafted as well. I finally volunteered for the United States Public Health Service, expressing my desire to work in Africa if possible. Several weeks later, after my papers had been processed through Washington, D.C., I received a telephone call from the director of a U.S. Public Health Service malaria research project in Uganda. He wanted to know if I had any interest in joining his team. This wasn't what I really wanted to do, so I didn't commit myself to it. I asked him to send me additional information. Meanwhile, I learned from one of my classmates that the U.S. Public Health Service's Center for Disease Control had been given responsibility for running a smallpox-eradication and measles-control program in nineteen western and central African countries. The program was being funded by the United States Agency for International Development.

This was more to my liking than the malaria research project. So I wrote to the center, expressing my interest in joining the program and telling them that my papers were already being processed for a commission in the Commissioned Corps of the U.S. Public Health Service. I received a telegram back from a Dr. Norris, who as head of the center's Smallpox Eradication Unit was in charge of the program. The next day he called me by phone.

"We're very interested in you," he said. "With your background and training you're ideal for one of the French-speaking countries."

CHAPTER 7

THE EPIDEMIC INTELLIGENCE SERVICE

When I flew away from a sizzling New York City heat wave on July 4, 1966, for Atlanta, Georgia, I had no idea of what lay ahead of me in the orientation program at the Center for Disease Control. The center, known by the acronym CDC, is located in the Druid Hills suburb of Atlanta, a short distance from Emory University. It's the hub of America's medical intelligence network, the nerve center where reports of epidemics are received and from where teams of disease fighters are quickly dispatched to control epidemics all over the world.

"It was typhoid in January, cholera in February, bubonic plague in March, typhus in April, smallpox in May and yellow fever in June," said the speaker who began the orientation course. "We're called to all parts of the world, India, Africa, South America and even the Arctic." The dead silence which filled the pauses between his statements gave great drama to what he said.

"You are now Epidemic Intelligence Service Officers, the cream of the crop, men who have been selected through a rigorous process. You are the new blood in an elite corps which has served with distinction all over the world."

There were seventy of us in the audience, young and enthusiastic physicians, mostly just out of internship and now being prepared for two years of service as medical detectives. Most would serve in the Epidemic Intelligence Service Corps, assigned to local health departments throughout the United States. A few would remain on at the center in special programs. Within the audience was a small group of us who were going to Africa to run the Smallpox Eradication and Measles Control Program. We were officially called "Smallpox Eradication Program Officers" while the rest were known as "Epidemic Intelligence Service Officers." It was an administrative distinction without much significance. Although our training would be the same, our experiences would be vastly different. The epidemic problems of Africa were markedly unlike those of California, New York and Iowa!

The speaker went on. "To carry out our mission we have had to stop ships at sea, intercept aircraft in the air and get the rapid decisive support of NATO and the Congress."

We sat glued to our chairs. I sensed a surge of excitement not just inside myself but throughout the audience. All of this exceeded my wildest fantasies.

"You will rescue cities from epidemics, save children from the ravages of disease and prevent sickness and death from sweeping across the heartland of America." After he said this, the speaker, a short, thin nervous man in a black and white military uniform, announced that the Surgeon General of the United States Public Health Service was going to speak to us from Washington, D.C.

"Gentlemen," he said, "the Surgeon General." I almost stood up. So did a number of the others. The auditorium filled up with a lot of deafening static. The speaker motioned to some technicians to adjust the equipment. The static continued. He cocked his head, hopeful of hearing the Surgeon General's voice. Nothing.

"Gentlemen, we seem to be having some difficulty with the audio equipment. Turn it off," he ordered, waving to the technicians. "I know the Surgeon General would have wanted to welcome you aboard and tell you what an important mission you have ahead of you. Why, only a few weeks ago when I was with him at the White House, he told me how he was looking forward to speaking to you."

The Surgeon General never did get through to us, and I had no way of knowing that a year and a half later I would be traveling with him in Mali, showing him the operations of the Smallpox Eradication and Measles Control Program.

The Epidemic Intelligence Service Course was a six-week-long program in which we were taught epidemiology and biostatistics. I had just completed similar course work of much greater length at Tulane. By the end of the first week, I realized that the epidemiologic principles and problems were the same. And the course in biostatistics was taught by my former professor from Tulane!

"I've been through all of this before," I said to one of my superior officers. "Can't I do something other than take the course?"

He was understanding, but there was nothing he could do about it. So I had to take the course.

While most of the physicians were just out of their internships, a few like myself had completed residency training in either internal medicine or pediatrics. Only a few had been through schools of public health. So for the majority, the course presented concepts not generally stressed in medical school. But learning concepts, as I had done at Tulane, didn't strike me as sufficient preparation to change someone into a medical detective. Even the best six-week wonders couldn't tackle most of the problems we learned about. And our instructors, like my professors at Tulane, stressed that medical detectives were really made through the process of wearing out a lot of shoe leather. So ahead of us lay a period of apprenticeship in which we would chalk up experience under the guidance of older and more seasoned epidemiologists. Most of the men assigned in the United States would receive that kind of guidance. But those of us who would go out to Africa would later find ourselves pretty much on our own.

"How are you going to do it?" I asked my roommate Bill Johnson as he packed up his things, preparing to leave for his assignment to a state in the Midwest.

"Darned if I know just yet. I guess I'll just have to handle whatever comes up with a lot of fast shuffling and fancy guesswork."

"But suppose it's something you're not sure of, a way-out kind of disease," I said.

"I'll just think of zebras, like the boss said."

Those of us who were going to Africa had to wait at the Center for several more months until final arrangements were made for our departure. During that time we were given an extensive course in smallpox eradication and one in French.

A few weeks after he left, Bill wrote to say that it wasn't that tough after all, though sometimes he was just one step ahead of everyone else or had to read up on the disease as he flew to the site of the outbreak. He tracked down an epidemic of food poisoning in a high school and found the source to be a sweet old lady who prepared food in the cafeteria. She was a healthy carrier. He couldn't allow her to continue working there, but he was able to get her transferred to the library! That stopped the epidemic!

Like many other young epidemiologists, Bill worked under the supervision of a local public-health epidemiologist, some of whom trained at CDC. By the end of two years he acquired enormous experience as a shoe-leather epidemiologist and became very expert because of the good supervision he had and also because he got involved in a number of interesting and difficult disease outbreaks. And then he left to start a residency in internal medicine in preparation for going into private practice. "What a loss," I moaned, after reading his letter in Africa. Bill wasn't an exception to the rule. Every year most of the Epidemic Intelligence Service Officers leave to go into residency training or else into positions in private practice, medical centers, research institutes or administration. It's a terrible loss of talent, one that has been going on for many years.

Most physicians are clinically oriented; they like caring for sick people. And that holds true for many who enter the Epidemic Intelligence Service. Two years of epidemiology and they're ready to go back to clinical medicine, not because they don't like epidemiology, but because they prefer treating patients. And the fact is, the private sector in medicine offers incredibly better remuneration, greater freedom and independence, denied to those in government service. Contrary to popular belief, there is little to attract physicians to government service, where most of the positions in epidemiology are found. The starting salary for a physician working full time in a hospital emergency room is almost double that of a trained epidemiologist who starts working for a health department. Federal, state and city government health agencies can't pay epidemiologists more because they are paralyzed by all sorts of civil service regulations which place limits on salaries. Naturally the law of the marketplace exerts a strong influence, the end result

88

being that epidemiologists are eventually drained off into more attractive and financially rewarding careers.

"It's great being an epidemiologist," Bill said to me after he quit, "but I can't support my wife and two kids on the salary." His words had little impact on me because I was still a bachelor living overseas in U.S. Government quarters. Three years later, after I returned to the United States, I understood what he was talking about. Unfortunately, the disadvantages of being an epidemiologist far outweigh the professional rewards as one grows older and acquires family responsibilities. That's why most of the CDC epidemiologists who are interviewed on television, the radio and in the papers seem so young.

When Bill left for the airport that day for his assignment out West, it didn't dawn on me that within a few years he and most of my Epidemic Intelligence Service Course classmates would give up epidemiology as a life career. This loss, which continues, is like spilling vintage wine just when it has mellowed and aged.

There are many rewards though, not all intangible either.

About these, there is more to come!

CHAPTER 8

THE HOT DRY WIND

By the end of two years in Mali, I had moved with the vaccination teams across almost thirty thousand square miles of rolling hills, wooded valleys, flood plains and sand dunes and had vaccinated close to three million people against smallpox and a million children against measles. No smallpox cases had occurred in the country in almost a year and I was flushed with a sense of success.

Now I led the teams into little-known country along the headwaters of the Bani River. It was still an isolated corner of Mali covered with velvety grasslands and dense woodlands full of herds of roan antelope and some of the last remaining elephants in the country. Here and there were villages, and spreading out from them along the river, patches of cultivation. People here grew corn, millet and rice and kept small herds of cattle, sheep and goats.

My two years in Mali had thus far been a great and adventurous challenge, because besides investigating epidemics of smallpox and measles, I had also come to know many diverse and extraordinarily interesting peoples. To some degree I had learned to see with their eyes and to understand their view of life. Their world was full of gods and spirits who traveled on the wind and moved along the bottom of the rivers. People knew the haunts of these spirits and believed that their anger or joy played an important role in people's fate. A lot of people in Mali were Moslem, but interestingly, they hadn't given up many of the practices associated with their old animist cults. Men prayed at the mosque, but they also made sacrifices in secret to their ancestors. In the region along the Bani River, the old animist spirits had become Moslem genies who haunted the mountain tops and the bottom of wells. The Moslems believed that God and all these spirits and genies as well as those shamans who could control their powers started epidemics, caused disease and healed the sick.

I had learned early on to present vaccines as talismans that ward off evil spirits and not as biological agents which stimulate antibodies which destroy viruses. This approach worked in most places, but not everywhere. Ideally, I should have educated people about the functions of vaccines. I was more than willing to do so, but health education in Africa will take years to accomplish, years which I didn't have at my disposal. And I wasn't patronizing these people in any way by using their own beliefs to bring them better medicine. There was much in their own indigenous medical therapies which I found to be of value. They managed most psychiatric patients very well, placing them in a structured supporting family environment which often brought about a quick remission of neurotic disorders. And from what I could judge, many of their herbs were effective. I spent a great deal of my spare time when I was out in the bush studying traditional medical beliefs and practices and later wrote a book on the subject which was entitled *African Folk Medicine*. These studies brought me into close contact with all sorts of healers and opened for me a treasure chest of knowledge.

It was easy going along the river. Most people lived within reach along the banks. I wondered if I hadn't made a mistake in extending my tour in Mali for another two years. Smallpox was almost wiped out, and in another year the whole country would be vaccinated. Because things were going so well, I decided to go back to Bamako for a few days' rest.

I started back early in the morning, before sunrise. The early-morning air in this part of Africa is cool and scented, an unexpected surprise in a dry and arid corner of the world. The woodlands swept by me, a collage of tall silk cotton trees, enormous baobab giants and sturdy-looking shea butter trees. There was a slight chill in the air, but as soon as the sun pushed itself up over the horizon, the chill and scents disappeared, whisked away by the dry hot air.

It was only during the rainy season and in the predawn hours that nature opened her beauties in Mali. I loved the rainy season for its sweet-smelling grass, flowering shrubs and enormous clear horizons full of blue skies and giant white puffy clouds. Toward late afternoon, thunderstorms would race across the distant skies, great swirling masses of black clouds streaked with lightning. At other times of the day, a soft drizzle would fall from a patch of gray sky, surrounded by rays of sunshine.

My truck, bouncing along the track at forty miles an hour, made so much noise that it seemed the bush was full of silence. But whenever I stopped, the sounds of life rushed in on me. I could hear the travels of a nearby stream, the gentle conversation of village life and the songs of birds drifting through the trees. The dry season filled this land with a desiccated harshness and deprived nature of her ability to bring forth all of her magnificent reserves. The rains had ended four months before and now the blue skies and white clouds were replaced by a dense horizon of dust and heat waves. The harmattan had started blowing down from the Sahara, a dry hot wind full of dust and sand which covers this part of Africa for several months beginning in December. This year it seemed worse and it felt hotter to me than the two dry seasons I had already spent in Mali. It was going to be another four months before the wet monsoon would blow off the Atlantic and drive the hot dry air back into the Sahara. Four months is a long time when it's 120 degrees Fahrenheit in the shade at ten in the morning.

When I got back to Bamako, I took a shower to wash off the dust and to lower my own body temperature so that I wouldn't feel like a torn-up dishrag. And then I rushed down to my office which was in the compound of the Hygiene Service. Nowadays I would probably stretch out in bed in an air-conditioned room, thinking it a well-deserved compensation after traveling five hundred miles in the heat. But I was younger then.

My office was a small cubicle about ten feet square. The walls and floor were made of cement and the furniture was gray metal U.S. Government issue. The red dust built up in layers on everything. Even the leaves on the trees were covered with it. And people coming in from long road trips had red hair and eyebrows. The only way to clean the office was to wash it down with a hose— walls, furniture and floors. Eight years later when I was Commissioner of Health of New York City with an enormous office with oak paneling from floor to ceiling and wall-to-wall carpeting, I used to think back to my Bamako office and shake my head in disbelief.

During the time I lived in Bamako, it was a city of close to two hundred thousand people, built mostly of mud-brick houses. The small European community, which numbered less than five thousand, lived in cement block houses. My house was a small three-room bungalow with cement walls, a red terra-cotta roof and tiled floors. It was spartan and spare, as were the houses of other Americans in Bamako. But in a relative sense it was luxurious compared to the squalid conditions under which most of the Malians lived. Bamako was then a mosaic of unpaved streets, dust, open sewers, crowded noisy markets and herds of livestock. The air was acrid and polluted by the smoke of thousands of cooking fires. The hills behind Bamako blocked the flow of air so that by morning a thick white smog lay over the city. Where the Europeans then lived along the Niger River there were tall silk cotton trees and occasional cool breezes. But the rest of the town was hot and dusty, squalid and harsh. I never knew the meaning of abject poverty until I came to Bamako. For in East Africa, although people were poor, the ones I saw lived in cleaner and more open conditions and were happier and healthier than the crowded masses of Bamako.

I was lucky in that my work took me out of Bamako at frequent intervals. It wasn't a pleasant place to live. There were no new buildings such as those then going up in coastal Dakar and across the continent in Nairobi. Whatever the French had built was slowly falling into decay. For the Europeans and Americans who lived in the city, life was hard compared to what they were accustomed to back home. This wasn't the case in many other African capitals where expatriates had homes and a standard of living they could never afford in their homeland. This physical hardship was compounded by the oppressive Marxist regime then in power and by the lack of consumer goods in the markets. Bamako's only large grocery store carried nothing but Russian mustard and Polish beer for most of 1968. Mali's then near financial collapse, enormous external debt and unwise economic policies resulted in scarcities for everyone, for Malians themselves as well as for Europeans and Americans. The latter were able to deal with this by ordering canned goods and consumer items from the diplomatic export houses in Denmark. But the Malians had to suffer their privations in silence. Eventually the situation changed after the military coup which took place in late 1968. More liberal policies were adopted, resulting in the appearance of consumer goods back on the market.

The greatest challenge to Americans living in Bamako wasn't the heat or the air pollution or the filth, but the grinding boredom of the place. There was simply nothing to do. The existence of travel restrictions imposed by the Malian Government coupled with the poor roads and lack of decent accommodations for travelers out in the bush effectively prevented most foreigners from leaving Bamako.

Previous groups of American diplomats had devised ways of coping with this problem. Their legacy to those who followed was an institutionalized program of social activities. People invited one another to dinner at frequent intervals; swim lunches lasting from ten in the morning to three in the afternoon were held on Sundays at one of the four swimming pools in the American community and cocktail parties were thrown every several days to mark either someone's arrival or departure. The embassy showed current American movies one night a week on the ambassador's lawn. There were several local movie houses in Bamako, but they showed films made in India and poor-quality westerns made in Spain by Italian film companies.

Making meaningful social contacts with Malians in Bamako was difficult, a far cry from the situation in rural villages. Many of the educated Malians who lived in Bamako had been conditioned by a regimented catechism of Marxism and saw a plot behind every social gesture. They took satisfaction in being discourteous to Americans. It wasn't unusual that Malians simply didn't show up when invited by the American ambassador to social affairs. Some were afraid to come because of Mali's official anti-American policies. But for others it was an opportunity to show their contempt for America.

In looking back, I think that the Americans who lived in Bamako at that time—and there were about fifty of us—did rather well and made the best of a situation which was both difficult and unpleasant. A number, including myself, became interested in African art. The steady spread of Islam had led to the abandonment of traditional cults and the art objects associated with them, so Bamako was full of masks and statues, some of which were quite old. It was a collector's paradise, rendered easy by the fact that the merchants who sold these objects came to the houses of foreigners during lunch and at dinner time. The market was also full of a number of recently sculpted objects which I collected as well.

It was easy to fill in the slow hours of an empty evening negotiating the price of a mask with a merchant. Bargaining could sometimes take hours, conducted with great civility by both parties, in between which there were discussions about family, friends and the weather. Americans who collected would show their recent acquisitions to others, which provided another opportunity to fill in spare time.

My interest in ethnography was added to my interest in collecting African art in Mali through a peculiar twist of circumstances. When I returned from East Africa in 1962, I sent photographs of some of Martin and Osa Johnson's old campsites to Osa's mother, Mrs. Belle Leighty. At the time I didn't know whether she was still alive, but I sent them anyway, to the town of Chanute, Kansas, where I knew Osa and her family once lived. What a delight it was when two weeks later I received a reply from Mrs. Leighty. She told me that the town of Chanute had recently erected a museum in honor of her late daughter and son-in-law in which all of their memorabilia was exhibited. In 1964, I visited the museum and delivered a lecture on my experiences in Kenya and Tanganyika. During that visit, Mrs. Leighty showed me an unfinished manuscript which Osa had written, describing the last trip she and Martin took together. It was to Borneo in 1935. She asked me to take it to New York and try to get it published. The book was finally accepted by a leading publisher on the provision that I finish it, which I did using Osa's diaries and letters. It was called *Last Adventure* and released in 1966. This was a fantastic experience for me, to edit the last journey of my old boyhood hero and heroine! Soon thereafter I was made a trustee of the museum and became active in its affairs.

When I knew that I would be going to Mali, I held lengthy discussions with the directors of the museum about setting up a hall of African art. They were enthusiastic about the idea, but the museum lacked the funds to purchase the necessary objects. I then decided to collect objects myself which would later be used in the museum's hall.

Since I spent so much time out in the bush, I was able to observe people using masks in those villages where ancient beliefs were still strong. But I made it an unbreakable rule never to collect art objects in the bush, only in Bamako, as it held potential for souring my relationship with villagers who still held them sacred and could have negative effects on my medical program. But villagers were delighted to share their knowledge of the meanings and uses of art objects and I spent the long hours of most evenings in the bush collecting this kind of information and data on traditional medical beliefs and practices. I filled many lonely hours in Bamako writing up these studies which were later published in a number of professional journals. I also documented the use of many masks on film, taking thousands of photographs of them. As an amateur photographer, I also photographed the Malian landscape, people, customs, the seasons and the periods of the day. Thinking back now, I filled what could have been a burdensome and lonely void with a variety of available interesting activities. In 1974, the Martin and Osa Johnson Safari Museum opened the Hall of African Culture, which contains close to two hundred objects which I collected in Africa. It is the largest permanent exhibition of African art in that part of the country and one which I later donated to the museum.

Whatever spare time I had in Bamako—and there was very little as I recall—was taken up by my serving as physician to the American community. I was then the only American physician in the country, so my services were very much in demand. I treated people for a variety of minor and serious problems and not infrequently had to request their evacuation to a military hospital in Germany. The problems I dealt with in Bamako included kidney stones, hepatitis, appendicitis, broken limbs and fractured skulls, malaria, dysentery and psychiatric disorders. The embassy nurse, Maxine Bradrick, who came from California, arrived in Bamako several months after me and stayed on for more than ten years. We also managed the medical problems of visiting tourists. There weren't many who came to Mali in those days. But those who did were usually older people past retirement who often had chronic heart, circulatory and lung disease. Not infrequently we had to make house calls to Bamako's small hotels to care for these people when they became ill.

Two days after I arrived back in Bamako from the Bani River, a six-year-old boy named Diabie Traore was brought into the compound of the Hygiene Service. He had meningitis. I saw him from my desk, laid out on a blanket on the veranda just outside my office. His mother stood anxiously nearby, clutching her veil. I went out to look at him. He was such a pathetic sight, lying there on the ground. I didn't have any doubts that he had meningitis, nor did the chief nurse who was examining him. He had a high fever, a stiff neck and was semicomatose.

Some of the old French colonials had been saying for weeks that it hadn't been so hot and dusty in years, that it was epidemic meningitis weather. I hope to God there isn't going to be an epidemic, I thought. It would be a hellish job to control it in a place like Bamako.

Diabie Traore developed a fever and then a headache and was taken to the local dispensary. The nurse was alert and made the diagnosis. All cases of communicable diseases in Bamako were generally sent to the compound of the Hygiene Service which operated the lazaret out on the edge of town. When I first came to Bamako I was astonished that they had a lazaret. Lazarets were first established in Europe during the Middle Ages as places for the isolation of people with leprosy and later on for the isolation and treatment of people with other communicable diseases. They were named after Lazarus, the poor beggar with leprosy who lay at the gate of the rich man in one of Christ's parables in the New Testament.

The lazaret on the edge of Bamako functioned like one from the Middle Ages. It consisted of a few squalid cement buildings with tin roofs. There was one faucet with running water, no electricity and no beds. Medical treatment was summary and nursing nonexistent. The Hygiene Service and the lazaret were directed by an old Malian doctor whose other functions included mosquito and fly control and handing out summonses to people who threw garbage and dirty water into the already incredibly filthy streets. Dr. Sougoule was about as incompetent as they came. He spent most of his time hearing cases in his office. People would come in to protest against the summonses a horde of undisciplined so-called sanitary inspectors handed out. The usual victims were women, charged with throwing dirty water into the street. The streets were so filthy anyway, I thought they did a service to the city by watering down the microbe-loaded dust.

98

The women came with a retinue of shouting relatives and bribes in the form of money and chickens. It was worth their effort to argue the cases because the fines ran about a week's salary, on the average. My office was five feet away from this turbulent scene and over the years I also heard several thousand cases. Sougoule also held office hours and it wasn't unusual to see him sitting behind his desk examining someone with his stethoscope. The fully clothed patients bent over the desk top to get within reaching distance of the stethoscope.

Diabie Traore was loaded onto a pickup truck, the same one that Sougoule used for hauling produce from his farm nearby. They drove him out to the lazaret. I watched the truck move out through the gates and down the hot dusty road. I worried about his uncertain fate.

Sunday was a holiday and no one worked at the Hygiene Service except one male nurse who was on duty to give vaccinations. I usually went in for an hour or so late on Sunday mornings to clear up the paper work, do the filing and the typing. Secretaries were as rare as jukeboxes in Mali so I had to do most of this work myself.

"Bon jour, Docteur." Dionke Kaladioula, the nurse, bowed and salaamed in the doorway.

"Bon jour. Ça va chez toi?" I said looking up from the typewriter keyboard.

He hesitated, wrung his hands a little and then stammered out with a statement that all wasn't well. Malians were never candid about bad news. They led up to it in polite gradual steps, cushioning every phrase with euphemisms.

Dionke was tall and lean, quiet and strong inside. He switched from French to Bambara, the lingua franca in Bamako. He felt more comfortable with it, better able to use metaphors and circumlocutions.

"I wish that all was well, but Allah has wished it otherwise. It is that way in the affairs of men. We are on this earth for such a short time and we must accept Allah's will in all things."

Dionke's speech rambled on through lofty heights and was far better than the sermon I had heard earlier in the morning at the Catholic church.

"Allah is great," he pronounced with solemnity and reflection.

"Yes, Allah is great," I said. "What has he done now?"

99

Dionke pondered, shifted from one foot to the other and stared out into the quiet compound. The flamboyants were in bloom, massive umbrella trees, a deep fiery red.

"You see what he can do?" Dionke stared off at the flamboyants. "And there," he added, pointing up to the towering tops of the silk cotton trees. The branches were covered with rows of huge fruit-eating bats which migrated to Bamako each year at this time. They hung lazily in the sun. "You see how they come here every year."

"Yes, Dionke," I said a bit impatiently. "Allah is great and he has made all of these things. But what did he do today that he didn't do yesterday?"

"This morning when I came here four people from Bozola arrived with meningitis. I sent them in the Land-Rover to the lazaret."

"Did you tell Dr. Sougoule?"

"No, he was nowhere to be found."

"Are you sure it's meningitis?"

"I think so. What else could it be? They had stiff necks, headaches and fever."

There wasn't a telephone at the lazaret and I couldn't go there on my own without being asked to. The Malians were still sensitive about that sort of thing even though the old Marxist regime of President Modibo Keita had been overthrown in a coup d'etat in November of 1968, two months before. The new military government was somewhat more liberal about most things, but standard operating procedures put into place by the old government still ran the day-to-day affairs of the bureaucracy.

I was really worried now about an epidemic. Four new cases in the same quarter of the city was an ominous sign. I couldn't say for sure that an epidemic would happen. The next few days would tell the story. But my detective instincts told me that something big was unfolding. Something's got to be done, I kept thinking. I've got to alert the minister of health and the director general of health. I tried to track them down by phone, but they weren't at home.

"No one's around." I grimaced at Dionke, still standing patiently in the doorway, meditating his own thoughts.

"We will have to wait until tomorrow," he said softly. "Allah willing, nothing more will happen."

Dionke shuffled off the veranda and around to the front of the building and his small vaccination station.

I pondered what to do. Perhaps I was overreacting. Malians took calamities in stride. Thousands could die and they would accept it with graceful fatalism, undermining any confidence they might have about altering what they perceived as the inevitable God-ordained course of events. So talking to the minister and director at this point wouldn't serve much purpose, I concluded.

I decided to drive over to see Dr. Jean Duval, a pediatrician from Réunion Island, who had been directing Mali's maternal and infant health service since the early 1960s. Jean was bright, conscientious and dedicated and Mali was lucky in having someone like him. He was the only pediatrician in the country at the time. He never got any rest, even at night and on holidays. Children were brought to his house in a never-ending stream. He was so dedicated he took care of them on his own time, without ever receiving a fee.

We had become very close friends and colleagues and, lucky for me, have remained so to this day.

We exchanged pleasantries and I told him what had happened over the past two days at the Hygiene Service.

"Five cases is far too many in two days." He looked grave.

"That's what I thought," I said.

"And they're all in the same part of the city?" he asked.

"Over in Bozola."

"So they're clustered geographically," he replied.

"Clustering's occurred and obviously spread and that's what has me worried. You know," I said, "we're not going to be able to tell if a pattern is emerging until tomorrow or the day after. But the minister should start making some sort of plans now."

Jean was wiser and more experienced. "Too early to expect that. You know how things move here. The important thing is that you've picked up on something that has potential for being a very big epidemic. But it hasn't happened yet. We've got to watch it very closely. If there's a sharp rise in cases, the minister has to move fast."

I couldn't wait to get down to the Hygiene Service the next morning. When I drove my big Dodge truck through the gate, the compound looked the same as it did any other morning. But the morning itself was to be very different.

Dr. Sougoule was extremely agitated when he arrived. I supposed he was upset about the meningitis cases.

"You know about the meningitis cases that came in yesterday," I said.

"No, what cases?"

"The four from Bozola."

"Hmm, four cases. Nothing to worry about. They always get meningitis in that part of town."

What an idiot he was, making light of the whole thing.

"Are you going to the lazaret this morning?" I asked.

"No, I can't. That specimen of an imbecile Kouyate closed Habib's Pastry Shop yesterday without authorization and I have a hearing in a half hour."

At that point Kouyate came in. He was a young sanitary engineer who had just returned to Mali after studying for several years in France. He was bright, eager and honest.

Sougoule got up from behind his desk. "You damn fool!" He waved his finger in Kouyate's face. "How dare you close down that shop."

"It's a pigpen. I've never seen such a filthy place in my life," Kouyate shouted back.

"What's so filthy about it?"

"Haven't you ever seen where they make their pastries in the back? They have a latrine in the center of the room where they mix the dough." Kouyate made a circular motion with his arms outlining the latrine. "The workers defecate in the latrine and wipe their asses with their fingers and some water from a teapot. Then they wash their fingers off with a little water and go back to making pastries."

"What's wrong with that?" Sougoule demanded angrily.

"What's wrong? Don't you realize their fingers are full of microbes?"

"They wash them, don't they?"

"Wash? I don't call that washing. They just spread the germs around all over their hands. There should be a sink with hot running water and they should wash their hands thoroughly."

Habib's was a popular shop in Bamako, especially with the French. Their pastries looked tantalizing, displayed on elegant doilies in refrigerated cases. Some were smothered with cream and chocolate and others stuffed with fruit fillings. Out in front was a cozy sidewalk café where French women liked to sit in the late afternoon and nibble at both the pastries and at Bamako's petty gossip. According to Kouyate, they and the others who ate the pastries took in a big dose of microbes as well. Smothered in with the cream, chocolate and fruit fillings were probably bacteria such as the one which causes typhoid fever.

"I've been eating stuff from that shop for twenty years and I've never gotton sick." Sougoule's claim carried no weight with Kouyate.

"Just because you never got sick doesn't make the place sanitary and safe."

The two men argued and the argument grew more intense once Habib and his enormous entourage of character witnesses, friends, relatives and workers arrived on the scene. Sougoule had already made up his mind to reverse Kouyate, and I suspected that he had cut a deal with Habib. But he was skilled enough to know that he had to go through the charade of a hearing and listen to both sides of the story.

While this was going on a truck arrived in the compound from the Bozola dispensary. I didn't see it when it pulled in. But Dionke knocked on the window behind my chair and said, "There are fifteen people with meningitis!"

I broke into Sougoule's hearing and told him what was outside. The patients were being placed on the ground in front of the veranda leading to his office.

"Hmm, looks like more cases of meningitis." He shouted to an assistant. "Take them to the lazaret."

Facing the audience again he said, "How deep is this latrine?"

I couldn't believe it. This idiot was talking about a latrine and a pastry shop and outside were fifteen people with meningitis. Some were almost in coma, others curled up with muscle spasms, and now they were being trucked off to the lazaret while he talked about pastries! I wanted to smash his face in.

I picked up my phone and called Jean. "There are fifteen more cases!" I panted.

"Fifteen! My God! We've got the start of an epidemic!" he exclaimed.

"Get over here fast," he said. "We'll go up to Government Hill and see the minister."

It took me five minutes to get to Jean's office and another ten

103

from there to the top of Government Hill. He had called the minister, told him what had happened and that we were on our way. The minister, Dr. Benitieni Fofana, had been in office for about two months. He had studied medicine in France and was widely traveled. His director general of health, Dr. Daouda Keita, was also well trained and had a degree in public health from Montreal. I felt sure that given the facts, they would get things moving.

What I wasn't so sure of now was what to advise them. The truth was I knew very little about meningitis. The facts which raced through my mind were those I had picked up during my cram reading over the weekend. Before coming to Mali, I had seen only one case when I was a third-year medical student working on the pediatric ward at Kings County Hospital in Brooklyn, New York. The case was considered a zebra by the medical staff. Meningococcal meningitis was by then as rare as a hen's tooth in places like New York. The patient was a nine-year-old girl who had developed some of the severe complications of the disease, including damage to her vital adrenal glands. The professor gave each of us a prescription for a sulfa drug. "Take it for three days," he said. "Otherwise you might contract meningitis. You've all had close contact with the case."

That was it. The sum total of my personal experience with meningitis. Whatever else I knew I had read. We sped up the steep slopes of Government Hill toward the Ministry of Health. In my mind I rehearsed the little I knew. Meningitis is an inflammation of the coverings of the brain and spinal cord. These three delicate coverings are called the meninges. Meningitis can be caused by a variety of microbes, including bacteria, viruses, fungi or parasites and also by chemical agents. The kind of meningitis that had broken out in Bamako is known by a variety of names: cerebrospinal meningitis, cerebrospinal fever, spotted fever and meningococcal meningitis. The word cerebro refers to the brain and spinal to the spinal cord. The disease is caused by a tiny bacterium shaped like a double ball whose scientific name is *Neisseria meningitidis*. This microbe can live in the noses and throats of healthy people and cause absolutely no illness at all or perhaps at most a mild sore throat. Such people act as healthy carriers and spread the microbe to other people who like them may also become carriers for a while. But in some of them the microbe invades the lining of the nose and throat and enters the bloodstream. From there it spreads throughout the body, causing chills, fever and body aches and pains. Some patients develop red spots on their skin at this time and that's why the disease has sometimes been called spotted fever, not an especially good term and one which is often confused with other diseases which have the same name.

The microbe can continue to circulate around in the bloodstream for weeks and even months if not destroyed by antibiotics. But in most people the microbe leaves the bloodstream quickly and invades the coverings of the brain and spinal cord. People develop headache, backache, fever, chills, vomiting and a stiff neck.

Meningococcal meningitis occurs in the United States as well as in other parts of the world, though only a small percentage of people who come into contact with the microbe get meningitis. For this reason, cases in the United States tend to occur haphazardly and occasionally rather than in massive numbers. But epidemics have occurred in the United States in the past and as recently as in the 1960s in several U.S. Army camps where recruits were housed in crowded facilities. During those army-camp epidemics it was learned that crowding enhances the spread of the disease, especially in sleeping quarters. The closer people sleep together, the better the chances are of the disease spreading because the microbe is passed from the nose and mouth of a carrier to those nearby.

Army doctors found that the disease could be prevented and epidemics stopped just by widening the space between bunks in sleeping quarters. Other scientists in South America found that the reason children are more often affected by the disease is that they tend to sleep closer together in groups, especially in poor areas. African children sleep that way too, as many as a dozen all bunched together like the petals of a flower, with their heads in the center. During the night they cough, sneeze, and the mucus from their runny noses is easily spread. No wonder that meningococcal meningitis has always been thought of as a disease of children.

But there is something about meningococcal meningitis in Africa that's different from the disease anywhere else in the world. At intervals of seven to twenty years, massive epidemics spread across that hot strip of the continent that lies just to the south of the Sahara. This part of Africa is known to medical experts familiar with meningitis as the *"meningitis belt."* It stretches for six thousand miles from Senegal in the west to the Sudan in the east and passes through several countries including Mali, Upper Volta, Niger, Nigeria, Chad and Sudan. In this belt, the disease is severe, especially among children whose natural resistance and immunity levels are lower than those of adults. Seeing these children huddled in the dark hot corners of their huts, burning up with fever and convulsing, is a heart-rending sight. They quickly become dehydrated, then comatose and, within a matter of hours, die an agonizing death. Small wonder then that in Mali and other places people believe that sorcerers are responsible for the disease.

There were no records kept on meningitis epidemics in the belt prior to the colonial period, but since 1905 good data have been collected. In Mali epidemics swept through in 1905, 1921, 1937, 1944 and 1950. From Mali they spread with clockwork precision eastward into Upper Volta, then on to Niger, Chad and the Sudan. But since 1950 an as yet unexplained phenomenon has occurred. The big sweeping epidemics starting in the west and rolling east no longer appear. Instead, epidemics have been limited to more localized areas and occur at intervals which simply can't be explained.

When I first read all of this I wondered why there was such a thing as a *"meningitis belt"* and why epidemics took place the way they did. There were no ready answers, only theories. Some scientists maintain that rainfall exerts an influence either directly or indirectly on these epidemics. As a rule the epidemics appear during the long hot dry season, November through May. Temperatures are very high then, humidity low and the harmattan brings down a lot of dust from the desert. Some think that the hot dry air and the dust damage the mechanical defenses of the linings in the nose and throat and make it easier for the meningitis microbe to penetrate and gain access to the bloodstream, the first step toward its causing meningitis.

The old-timers were right, I thought. They knew what they were talking about when they said it felt like meningitis weather. Bamako was so hot and dry that everybody felt it. The ground was fertile for the little double ball to wreak havoc.

I pulled the truck to an abrupt stop in front of the Ministry of Health building. Even here on top of the hill, where there was always a breeze, it felt like a furnace. Not a leaf moved in the mimosas; the cicadas drilled their annoyance with the heat into the dust-filled air. For me these were ominous signs and I felt that ahead of us lay impending doom.

CHAPTER 9

A HUNDRED DAYS OF FEAR

The minister of health, Dr. Fofana, and the director general of health, Dr. Keita, knew much more about epidemic meningitis than I had given them credit for. And they had no hesitating doubts about what had to be done. Fofana decided to hold a strategy meeting later in the day with all his division chiefs, including Sougoule and representatives from the ministries of Defense and Interior.

What a peculiar experience it was. Suddenly I was being taken into the confidence of the minister of health and asked to participate in a policy meeting in a country where only two months before a Maoist-style cultural revolution held a firm grip. But all that had been swept away in a flash along with the eight-year-old Marxist regime of President Modibo Keita on November 19, 1968. The fourteen-man military junta which toppled Keita changed the internal atmosphere of Mali overnight. Gone was the Marxist rhetoric, the pervasive salutation "Comrade," the popular militia, political indoctrination sessions, collective farms and that corrosive xenophobia and paranoia which bitterly tarnished Malians' relationships with Americans.

But many elite Malians, of course, had been well schooled in Marxism-Leninism, both in Mali and in schools from Kiev to Prague. It replaced the animism of their ancient ancestors and the

107

Islam of their immediate forefathers and they espoused it with fanatical fervor. They were mostly young and took themselves very seriously even though their life experience was often flimsy. They staffed the ministries, taught in the schools and operated the country's nationalized industries and companies. They didn't abandon their views, but they did modify their comportment toward Americans out of instincts of self-preservation.

As for the military who had seized power, they inherited a country which was not only financially bankrupt but one whose prospects for future solvency were very dim. For out of its parched earth, Mali could only yield peanuts, shea butter and gum arabic. But the average Malian's expectations rose after the coup because he firmly believed that Mali's misery was due to the oppression of Modibo Keita and his Marxist henchmen. He had forgotten that when independence came in 1960, Mali's misery was then attributed to alleged colonial exploitation. It was always somebody else's fault. Never could they bring themselves to admit that Mali was just plain poor. They were too proud a people for that, a people a little too aware of their ancient history which modern bards sang of with eloquent hyperbole. In the end it could be said that they had nothing else but their pride.

Day One–Day Three

It was decided that Saturday, January 25, 1969, be considered Day One of the epidemic for purposes of keeping track of its course. We all knew that cases had probably occurred before, but we weren't aware of them. By this count we were now in Day Three of the epidemic.

Fofana came to the meeting with an administrative strategy which effectively assigned key roles to very able people and isolated Sougoule from critical functions. His assistants had drawn up a list of retired Malian doctors and nurses who would be asked to come in to work treating patients in the lazaret, bolstering the permanent staff there which was to be augmented with nurses from the hospitals. The buildings at the lazaret were too small to accommodate more than two hundred people. And accommodations had to be provided not only for patients, but also for one or two of their relatives who would cook for them and act as their individual nurses. Central kitchens and dietary services were not a feature of many African hospitals at the time.

"We won't have time to build permanent buildings," Keita said. "We'll have to put up temporary shelters made of straw mats."

I had seen those shelters before. The straw mats were five feet in length and width and made of plaited elephant grass.

"They'll be a fire hazard," I said. "There's no electricity out there. Most people will be using kerosene lamps. Suppose one tips over and the mats catch fire?"

Keita shrugged. "What else can we do?"

I couldn't answer him right away, but the thought of bringing in an army field hospital flashed through my mind. I didn't mention it. I didn't have the authority to make such an offer and would have to talk it over first with the American ambassador, Ed Clark. For the time being we went ahead on the assumption that most people would be housed in straw-mat shelters.

There were only three latrines at the lazaret and one faucet and no electricity. What a confluence of adverse conditions! I told Fofana that I would talk to the American ambassador and see if the United States could provide funds for expanding the water lines and for bringing in electricity. "But more latrines will have to be dug, and right away," I added.

"We'll do that," Fofana replied, marking his words with an up-and-down movement of his hands. "But we'll need water and electricity there, so whatever you can get for us from your government will be greatly appreciated."

Fofana announced that he was putting all diagnostic and treatment responsibilities under the direction of a Malian doctor, Angirou Pangalet. He was a very able man and one who had been through the two previous epidemics of meningitis in Mali. After he announced that, we got into a lengthy discussion about how to treat the patients. The standard treatment in Mali and most of French-speaking West Africa at the time was a single shot of a sulfa drug known as sulfadiazine. This drug killed the little double-balled microbe in a matter of hours, as did a number of other sulfa drugs and antibiotics. The Malians were used to administering sulfa drugs to cases of meningitis and met with success in over 95 percent of them.

"But they may be resistant to sulfa drugs," I said. A great deal

109

of panic had swept through medical circles in the United States in the early 1960s when epidemics of meningococcal meningitis broke out in military installations which didn't respond to sulfa drugs. The first of these occurred at the United States Naval Training Center in San Diego and the second at Fort Ord in Monterey County, California. Then epidemics broke out in several other military installations and the story was the same. The little double ball was resistant to sulfa drugs.

"I'm familiar with the Fort Ord experience," Keita said. That epidemic and the others which followed it were caused by Group B organisms. We have Group A here in West Africa."

"You can't be sure of that" I said. "We don't even know if it's meningococcus really."

"We haven't cultured it out yet, if that's what you mean," Keita replied. "But from the epidemiologic evidence it can't be anything but meningococcus."

My instincts told me that he was right, but my sense of scientific precision was uncomfortable at tackling a problem without knowing the organism and its characteristics for sure.

"All right," I said, "suppose for the sake of argument it's Group A. How do we know that it hasn't become resistant to sulfa like Group B?"

"It could happen," Keita replied, "but right now we don't have any evidence of it and until we do we have to assume it's sensitive to sulfa."

Maybe he was right. But maybe he was wrong.

The only way to find out was to culture the organism in the laboratory. The Laboratoire de Biologie in Bamako had facilities to culture the microbe, but they couldn't tell what group it was or whether it was sensitive or resistant to sulfa. This meant that specimens had to be sent out of the country and Fofana went on to say that he would send specimens to a laboratory in Marseille which specialized in studying meningococci.

I asked him for permission to send some specimens to the Center for Disease Control in Atlanta, Georgia. The French labs were notoriously slow in getting results back to Bamako and the Malians usually didn't press them for a quick reply. We just couldn't afford that kind of long wait, not when there was a possibility that we were after all dealing with a microbe which would turn out to be a zebra.

110

Fofana thanked me, but politely declined my offer. Mali's new government may have been friendlier to Western nations than its predecessor, but it was playing a balancing act between East and West. My simple offer was a variable in the overall equation, one on which Fofana clearly didn't want to decide without higher clearance.

"Prevention has to be given a top priority," Fofana said. "All close contacts of patients must receive sulfa."

This was standard practice for many years in the United States, but the San Diego and Fort Ord epidemics had demonstrated that this strategy no longer worked. Contacts taking sulfa as a preventive were not protected from getting meningitis when the organism was resistant to sulfa. This marked the end of an era, the era when meningococcal meningitis could be quickly and successfully treated with sulfa and contacts completely protected by it. Military doctors turned to the next logical thing—treating patients with other antibiotics to which the organisms were sensitive. That worked for those already ill, but what didn't work was giving those same antibiotics to contacts to protect them. None of the antibiotics tried proved to be an effective prophylactic against the microbe.

I told the group all of this when the minister touched on this subject. "And," I added, "the problem is not so much with people who have contact with patients with meningitis, but with those who have contact with healthy carriers."

The carrier rate could be enormous during an epidemic. In San Diego close to 70 percent of the naval recruits were found to be healthy carriers during the epidemic. Susceptible people who contract meningitis generally pick up the germ from a healthy carrier and not from someone who is sick with meningitis. This was one of the maddening things about trying to control an epidemic. How could we possibly tell who was a carrier in a city of two hundred thousand people? And supposing we did know who they were? Could we do anything about it? No.

"I don't think it will be very useful to give sulfa out to contacts," I said.

"We have to," said Jean. "We can't assume that we're dealing with a resistant organism yet. You're thinking too far ahead and about developments which don't exist yet as far as we know."

There was a lot of discussion about dust and how to control it. Everyone still believed that, as in the past, if it rained, the epidem-

111

ic would end quickly. "So let's hope it rains," became everyone's expressed wish. I was puzzled about the relationship between rain and the end of previous epidemics. Cause and effect or just coincidence?

Day Four

I went out to the lazaret with Keita to look over the facilities and procedures set up the day before.

Pangalet, the physician in charge, had things well in hand. To get to the lazaret you had to cross a narrow concrete bridge over the Farako River. Four soldiers guarded the bridge twenty-four hours a day to keep curious onlookers out. Patients were first brought into a triage room at the entrance of the lazaret where the diagnosis was either made or excluded on the basis of the history and a physical examination. This wasn't difficult because most cases were pretty far gone. All of those I saw that afternoon had stiff necks. I examined them as they lay on the examining table. I put my hand behind their heads and tried to bend them gently forward. Not only were their necks stiff, but the bending movement caused their legs to fold up toward their bodies. This is an important sign in the diagnosis of meningitis and is due to irritation of the spinal cord and nerves going to the legs.

"They don't come in right away." Pangalet put on a pair of gloves to do a spinal tap. Everyone admitted to the lazaret had to be tapped.

"Why not?" I asked, watching the nurses hoist a seven-year-old girl onto a high stool. She was naked, dazed and terrified. When they sat her down on the stool and bent her forward for the tap she screamed and urinated.

"Oh, well, you see, they go to the local healers first," Pangalet said. "Those good-for-nothings charge them an arm and a leg for their useless charms and herbs. Instead of getting better, the patients get worse. You've been around here long enough, Imperato, to know that when the patients get worse and die, the healer doesn't get blamed. They say it's God's will."

My eyes darted between the poor girl and Pangalet holding what

112

wouldn't have been considered a pediatric tap needle where I had trained. It was enormous.

"Isn't that needle too big?"

He was candid. "Of course it is. Get me a smaller one and I'll use it. This is all we've got."

I had done plenty of spinal taps as an intern and resident, but always on patients lying on a nice clean bed. I would have them curl up in fetal position so that their lower backs would be well exposed and then I would sterilize the area with several applications of an antiseptic solution and drape it with sterile towels. The important thing was to get the needle through the space between the vertebrae and into the spinal canal where the fluid is. I got into trouble a couple of times because the space was narrow and the spine twisted or curved. Poking around caused the patient a lot of pain, especially when I pushed the needle by accident into bone. And if bleeding occurred, it wasn't dangerous to the patient, but it screwed up the tap. The few drops of blood would mix with the spinal fluid when it finally started to drip out through the needle. Normally there isn't any blood in the spinal fluid. When you're making the diagnosis of meningitis and other conditions it's important to see if there are red and white blood cells in the fluid that shouldn't be there. So blood-contaminated fluid was useless in helping with the diagnosis. The tap would have to be repeated.

Pangalet took his needle and slipped it into the girl's back in a flash after a nurse wiped the area with Merthiolate. The fluid that came out into the tall thin test tube looked like cream.

"Pus!" I said as I gaped.

"What did you expect?" Pangalet smiled. "Send it off to the laboratory."

"Not like in the United States," said one of his nurses.

"Do you want to do one?" Pangalet asked.

"I'm not really used to doing them this way. It isn't that I can't do them—er, it's just that it's all different here."

"It'll broaden your experience," Pangalet said offhandedly. "Put on gloves. There are sterile needles in the tray."

He shouted to the assistants. "Set up the old man. I'm going down the hill to check on things in the ward."

"You're not going to leave me here alone?"

"Why not? Come on, you can do it. Everyone's always saying

113

you're the only specialist in internal medicine in Mali. You shouldn't need me around now, should you?" He smiled and swaggered off.

The old man was already up on the stool. Pangalet's assistants were enormous brutes, more like laborers than medical auxiliaries. One had a head lock on the old man and another had his legs pinned down from a squatting position. A splotch of red Merthiolate was already on his back. I looked down at the needle. God, was I terrified! The poor old guy was in agony enough. What if I missed and screwed it up? He would be hurt and so would my pride.

"You had better get going. It's drying up and there's flies here." The nurse held the tube ready for the fluid.

I pushed the needle in after palpating the space between the vertebrae with my finger. It slipped through right into the spinal canal. I breathed a sigh of relief. The creamy fluid, full of pus and microbes, spurted out under enormous pressure into the tube. "You'd better take off three tubes," said the nurse. "You've got to relieve all that pressure." By the time I started filling the third tube, the fluid dripped out slowly instead of spurting out.

Pangalet was back. "How did he do?" he asked everyone.

"Akagne n'kossobe—Very good," they said in Bambara.

"Why did you leave me alone like that?"

He laughed. "If I didn't think you could do it I wouldn't have let you even try. I knew you could do it, but you didn't. Now you know you can."

He put on another pair of gloves for the next tap. "By the way, that child Diabie Traore is fine. Should be able to go home in a couple of days. He's down in the first building."

Day Ten

Fifty-nine cases occurred, bringing the total to five hundred since the beginning of the epidemic. That was a hell of a lot of cases. The Laboratoire de Biologie had identified the organism. It was the meningococcus as we suspected. The Malian government didn't make any official announcements about the epidemic. Nothing came over the radio. Nothing appeared in the paper. But people knew. Word had spread all over the city that the dreaded *finyabana* had broken out in Bozola and that it was spreading.

Five hundred cases of meningitis in Bamako's two-hundred-thousand population was equal to twenty thousand cases in a city like New York with eight million people. It was staggering! In New York, even a vague report of a case of flu touches off an epidemic of interest on the part of TV, radio and the press. In Bamako, there was no official news, only rumors—rumors that were a far cry from reality. The French women at Habib's Pastry Shop reported thousands dying and an epidemic of malaria and bubonic plague going on at the same time! Maybe there were microbes in the pastries, but I suspected there was also a dash of spirits.

Day Twenty

Ninety-two cases came into the lazaret this day and twenty people died. Pangalet kept a large chart on the wall in his office at the lazaret with curves showing the daily number of cases, deaths, temperature, barometric pressure and rain. There hadn't been any rain yet. The curve showing the cases was saw-toothed in appearance and it was steadily going up. Close to twelve hundred cases had occurred and two hundred deaths, all of them in the eastern part of the city. During the previous week, the epidemic had spilled out from Bozola and Niarela into two adjacent quarters, Medina-Coura and Missira. Ominously, it had spread to the main market areas where tens of thousands of people congregated during the day in crowded and poorly ventilated conditions. There was nothing preventing it from moving into the bulk of the city which lay to the west, protected by a thin block-wide line of government buildings.

Day Thirty

On the average there had been sixty cases a day coming into the lazaret, but this day there were ninety-seven. I had done some calculations on the cases and discovered that 60 percent of them were among children less than fifteen years of age. During the previous ten days, the disease had moved into the western side of the city as we had feared. It was all over now, from one part of town to the other, and had spilled across the Niger River into the small settlements there.

Panic set in. Many Europeans sent their wives and children out of the country to Dakar and Abidjan or to Europe and some wealthy Malians did the same. The flights coming into Bamako from Europe were empty. The railroad cars coming from Dakar carried only a handful of passengers, a far cry from the thousands who usually traveled in even on the roofs and sides when there was no room inside. Malians stuffed cotton into their nostrils, bought talismans from local healers and prayed at the mosques.

Day Forty

Ninety-eight cases occurred and the average per day was running about eighty.

The Malian army began watering down the streets with cistern tanks to reduce the dust and Sougoule decided that instead of fining women for throwing water into the streets, he would encourage them to do it!

There were close to four thousand people out at the lazaret, housed in thirteen enormous straw-mat shelters. When Diabie Traore entered the lazaret there were less than a dozen people there. Keita and Pangalet told me that the fatality rate was running close to 20 percent and this had them worried. That was a sharp rise over the earlier 10 percent. They had also noticed that people who had been given sulfa as a preventive were coming down with meningitis anyway.

I went out to the lazaret myself and made rounds with them.

"Dehydration," I said on leaving the first shelter. "A lot of those kids are dehydrated. They need salts and fluid. It isn't meningitis that's killing them, but electrolyte imbalance."

"But some who come in early and get treated and are not dehydrated die anyway," Pangalet said.

116

"It's got to be something else. Didn't you say that some of those who got sulfa were getting meningitis anyway?"

"Yes, I noticed it this past week."

"Resistance?" queried Keita.

"Maybe. Did the laboratory in Marseille send back any reports yet?"

"No. It's been over a month."

I now saw my chance. The Malian government, which was still doing its political balancing act, had turned down my request to send specimens to the States. And they wanted nothing to do with a field hospital run by American military personnel.

"I could get some specimens to CDC in Atlanta. We'd have a reply in a week."

"Let me talk to the minister," Keita replied.

He did later that day and I got permission to collect several specimens of spinal fluid and send them off to CDC. But the Malians didn't want the field hospital. They said they could do it themselves.

Dehydration was certainly responsible for some of the increased mortality, but I suspected that the double-ball microbe had become resistant to sulfa. CDC would be able to tell us, but it would take a week to get their report.

Day Forty-five

I had sent a summary of the epidemic to the CDC a few days before outlining what was happening and got a reply from Dr. Louis Williams, a specialist in meningococcal meningitis. He suspected that at the outset of the epidemic most cases were caused by organisms sensitive to sulfa. But sulfa given out as a preventive to so many people had knocked out the sensitive strains and left behind those which were resistant to it. This meant that sulfa wouldn't work in treating people either.

The Malian government received an offer of a new experimental vaccine against meningitis from a pharmaceutical company in France. A number of scientists in Europe, Canada and the United States had been working for many years, developing a vaccine

117

against meningococcal meningitis. None of these vaccines had been perfected or field-tested enough to prove that they were effective. But it was worth the try. The Malians had done everything they could so far. Public assemblies were banned, theaters closed, sulfa given out, the schools shut down. What more could they do?

Day Fifty

There were one hundred and eight cases, the most recorded so far in a single day. Earlier in the morning I was in my office getting the vaccinators and jet guns ready for the antimeningitis vaccination program which was planned for the following week when the vaccine was due to arrive. A call came from Ed Clark, the American Ambassador.

"Pat," he said, "can you come over to the embassy? There's a cable for you from CDC in Atlanta about the spinal-fluid specimens you sent. It's in highly technical language and we can't quite understand it."

"Will be right there."

I raced over to the embassy. For weeks we had been waiting for the French laboratory to send a report. None had come. CDC had delivered in record time. At last we would know what was going on.

The message in the State Department cable came from Atlanta to our Bamako receiver via the huge station State operated in Liberia. It was written in what we used to call "cabalese," short staccato phrases stripped of articles, conjunctions and modifiers.

My eyes raced down the long message. It was a page and a half long:

> . . . results serologic grouping and testing four specimens meningococci . . . all four Group A. Specimen one minimum inhibitory concentration (MIC) of sulfadiazine 0.5 mg percent and zone 45 mm sensitive. Specimen two MIC 20 mg percent and zone 19 mm resistant . . . same specimen three. Specimen four MIC 0.5 mg percent and zone 47 mm sensitive . . .

"What does it all mean?" one of the embassy officers asked.
"It means we're dealing with both horses and zebras."

"Horses and zebras?"

"Yes, we've got both."

"I don't understand."

"It means that two of the specimens are sensitive to sulfa drugs as most expected. They're the horses. And two are resistant. They're the zebras."

"Ah, so that's it! The horses you expect. But not the zebras. I have to remember that and use it in diplomacy some way."

I called Keita and Fofana and told them that we had both horses and zebras on our hands. They knew what I meant right away. The whole treatment plan at the lazaret had to be changed. And furthermore, we had to stop giving sulfa to contacts.

Day Fifty-six

The number of cases per day fell down to seventy, from the high of a hundred and eight six days before. I had just returned from a forty-eight-hour trip to Dakar. A filling had fallen out of one of my back molars and I had developed a toothache. The only dentist in Mali had left with his family for Europe because of the meningitis epidemic and I had put up with the toothache for over two weeks. I couldn't put up with it any longer. A two-hour air trip and a distance of a thousand miles and I was in a dentist's office in Dakar. It took only a half hour for an x-ray and the filling. But I had to wait until the following day to catch the five A.M. flight back to Bamako.

There had been close to three thousand cases in Bamako and four hundred deaths. I didn't realize how used I had become to this calamity until I got back from Dakar and saw the empty stores and closed movie theaters and scores of people walking around the streets with cotton plugs in their noses. Many Europeans gave their African servants paid leaves; they were afraid they would contaminate them with meningitis.

"We've changed the treatment plan," Pangalet said when I met him out at the lazaret. "Chloramphenicol and penicillin in addition to sulfa."

"Has it had any effect on the fatality rate?"

"It certainly has. We're now down to about 7 percent, a lot better than the 20 percent we were running with sulfa alone."

119

"When are you going to start the vaccination program in the schools?" he asked.

"In a couple of days. Vaccine hasn't come in yet."

"Think it'll work?"

"Can't say. It's experimental. Maybe yes. Maybe no."

"Did you know that they've had five hundred cases in Ségou?" he asked.

"No, but I'm not surprised. Probably many more than that. We just don't know about it. People die in their villages and it's never reported."

"Tip of the iceberg, as you always say," Pangalet replied.

Day Sixty-one

The number of cases had fallen to forty a day. The chart on Pangalet's wall showed a case curve which was resembling a bell-shaped distribution more and more. The epidemic had peaked and was now slowly entering its final phase. And it hadn't rained yet. The double-balled microbe had moved through the Bamako population, coming into contact with most people. Some got meningitis, but most developed immunity. The number of susceptible people was shrinking and that's why the number of cases per day had grown fewer and fewer.

We started vaccinating thirty thousand schoolchildren with the vaccine from France after this downward trend started. If we had started before that trend we could have come to the erroneous conclusion that the vaccine slowed the epidemic down. As I saw it, most of the children being vaccinated were probably already immune through direct contact with the microbe over the previous month and a half. This didn't mean that the vaccine wasn't effective. But it did mean that we couldn't really appraise its effectiveness because we were vaccinating a population that was largely immune already.

Day Ninety

During the previous three weeks, the number of cases per day fell to about twenty. While the epidemic wasn't over yet, it was fast approaching its end. By the time it did end there were 6,712 cases in Bamako and 759 deaths, the equivalent of 270,000 cases and 28,000 deaths had the epidemic occurred in New York City. By anyone's standards it was a medical catastrophe.

It was to be a few more years before safe and effective anti-meningitis vaccines were developed. What a different course of events if we had had those vaccines then! As it was, the people of Bamako said to themselves and one another that the sorcerer had had his revenge. And the physicians who gathered around Dr. Fo-fana's conference table for a final meeting after the epidemic was over were wiser about meningitis. As men of science we all knew that meningitis is caused by a microbe and not by sorcerers. And yet some of us believed that the rains played a crucial role in stopping meningitis epidemics.

I explained to those at the meeting that the start of the rains was only coincidentally related to the ending of meningitis epidemics. The evidence in favor of a causal relationship had never been strong. Causal relationships can never be assumed, they must be proven.

As we spoke, clouds rolled across the skies; there were gusts of wind, thunder and lightning and then the rain fell. It fell in torrents. It was the first rain of the year. But it was coming too late for anyone to give it credit for stopping the epidemic. The epidemic ended because the vast majority of people in Bamako had built up an immunity to the double-balled microbe.

CHAPTER 10

THE APOLLO DISEASE

Toward the end of 1970, smallpox was eradicated in Mali. I had been in the country four years and had seen four million people vaccinated against the disease. The mass-vaccination program was over. But that didn't mean my job was done. I had to see to it that the two hundred thousand children born in Mali each year were vaccinated. Smallpox still existed in other parts of Africa and the world and as long as it did there was always the danger that it could be reintroduced into Mali. Getting to these children wasn't easy. They were scattered all over the country. The cost of sending mobile teams out over great distances merely to vaccinate these children was prohibitive. The U.S. Government couldn't afford it. And certainly the Malians couldn't.

I finally solved the problem by coming up with the idea of giving out smallpox vaccine to all the dispensaries around the country. There were close to four hundred of them. With vaccine and ice chests, the nurses could slowly vaccinate all the newborns in their districts without much trouble. This sounded a lot easier than it really was. It took a year to put the whole plan into effect. I calculated that at the end of that year my work would be finished in Mali and I'd return to the States.

In early 1970, we weathered the first epidemic of yellow fever to strike Mali in over twenty years. It and the meningitis epidemic tested the mettle of the Malian health system. What no one knew at the time was that a new, even deadlier epidemic disease was on its way into the heartland of West Africa. Epidemics like this didn't make the front-page headlines in the Western world but only appeared on the back pages as box inserts. The thousands of deaths didn't make much of an impact either. People were solidly jaded. Africa had become synonymous with violence, revolution, totalitarian repression, massacres and regimes which preached one thing at the United Nations and practiced the opposite as far as their own people were concerned. Africa may have been receiving technical and material assistance from the Western world, but not much in the way of sympathy.

For a number of years, large numbers of political refugees had been coming into Mali from neighboring Guinea which had a despotic Marxist regime. The quality of life had to deteriorate dramatically for Africans to leave their homes. Obviously, this had occurred in Guinea. In the summer of 1970, the steady flow of political refugees brought out a strange story, stranger than any of those they generally recounted about Guinea's president. These refugees said that there was a new disease in Guinea. It was called *"Apollo."*

"What a strange name," I said to Jean Duval one Sunday afternoon as we drank coffee on his veranda.

"It's strange all right," he said, "but Apollo means speed to the Africans. That's what those space flights signify to them more than anything else."

"But I wouldn't give the name of a space-flight series to a serious new disease."

"No." He laughed. "You would say it was a zebra."

A zebra it certainly was from the description Guineans gave— vomiting, diarrhea and death within a matter of hours.

"Can't be typhoid," I said. "Too fast for that."

Jean nodded his agreement.

"And the other diarrheas we have in this area aren't usually accompanied by vomiting," I said, "or by sudden death."

"Maybe you'll think I'm crazy," Jean interjected, "but I think it's cholera."

"Cholera! Here in Africa?"

"Yes, cholera."

"Can't be. There's never been any cholera in this part of Africa in recorded history."

"Why can't it be cholera?" he asked. "You're the one who's always telling us to think of zebras. Well, cholera is a zebra." He laughed.

"But if it's cholera, how on earth did it ever get to Guinea? The nearest cholera cases are two thousand miles away."

He shrugged his shoulders. "I've no idea. But as you always say, the zebras come from the most unlikely sources."

Jean's guess was a bit far-out even for me. I knew something about cholera, but not much. I hadn't paid much attention to it. It didn't exist in the United States and was the only epidemic horror covered in tropical-medicine books which was absent from Africa. I used to flip over that chapter in my books. The pictures accompanying them were usually of Indians washing in the Ganges. Mali was a long way from India. It was a zebra all right, but not one that had ever grazed on the fields of Africa.

When I went back and reread the chapters on cholera, I realized that the descriptions matched what the refugees were saying. But I had doubts—doubts about the accuracy of their descriptions and doubts about the possibility of cholera suddenly appearing where it never was before.

In August, Dr. Fofana learned that the Guinean Government requested the assistance of the World Health Organization with a diarrhea problem they had in the capital city, Conakry. A special team of experts flew to Conakry from Geneva, including two world experts on cholera. One of these men was a personal friend of Fofana's. They spent ten days in Conakry, a miserable tropical hole with soldiers and popular militia guards stationed at every intersection. The Guineans held the team incommunicado during their stay. We had no way of knowing what was going on. But the stream of refugees still told the same story. Diarrhea like water, and it killed in a matter of hours.

On August 26, the team left Conakry to return to Geneva. Their plane stopped in Bamako for an hour. We went out to meet them. One of the leaders of the team, Dr. Renaud, was a world authority on the disease.

"It's cholera," he told us. "The Guineans refuse to recognize it officially."

"How did it get there?" Fofana asked, incredulous.

"We're not sure. The Guineans wouldn't let us out of Conakry to do any epidemiologic studies. But we've got strong suspicions that it was brought in from the Soviet Union."

"What makes you suspect that?"

"There are a lot of Soviets working in Guinea and a lot of Guineans traveling back and forth from the Soviet Union."

Fofana had a questioning look.

"The Soviets had a big epidemic of cholera this year in the south. It came in from Iran and the Middle East. They've kept it quiet and we don't know how widespread the epidemic was. But it was a big one."

"So you think someone with cholera, either a Russian or a Guinean, came back to Guinea incubating the disease," Fofana said.

"Yes, and then they came down with it and infected other people. Now this is just my theory. Some of the other members of the team think it plausible that the disease came to Guinea from a merchant ship. Ships empty their latrines at sea and if there were an epidemic on shipboard, the seawater would get contaminated. We found the organism in the water all along Conakry's beaches."

"But how real do you think that possibility is?"

"I don't think much of it," Renaud said. "From what we found out, the disease started well inland and not along the coast. It came down to the coast from the interior of the country. If a shipboard epidemic contaminated the seawater around Conakry, cholera would have broken out there first and not in the interior."

"How bad is the epidemic?" Fofana asked.

"Very bad. But the Guineans have suppressed all information about it. The president signed a decree making it a crime to mention the word cholera. All cases are called diarrhea. And then he had big parades in Conakry while we were there, with people carrying banners denouncing cholera as a disease of the imperialists."

The president of Guinea, Sekou Toure, was popularly viewed by many Africans and Europeans familiar with the country as mentally ill. He didn't capture headlines like Idi Amin of Uganda, nor did Jean Bokassa of the Central African Republic, the one who made himself emperor and had a huge coronation ceremony in 1978. Toure had been around for a long time and the Africans thought of him as a crazed, cruel despot who preached Marxism. But the Western world ignored him. His backwater country wasn't of any great strategic interest, except to aluminum companies which mined Guinea's rich bauxite deposits.

"I told them that we would report the disease officially if they didn't. Their minister of health said that Toure would resign from WHO if we did that."

Guinea had resigned from so many other international organizations that it seemed to me almost irrevelant if it resigned from WHO too.

"So what do you plan to do?" Fofana asked.

"Report it as cholera. We have to. We found a thousand organisms in each millimeter of seawater along the beaches."

"That many!" Fofana gasped like the rest of us.

"Yes and it's just a question of time before the disease moves up and down the coast to Sierra Leone, Liberia, Ivory Coast, Gambia and Senegal."

"Will it come inland?"

"Can't say."

"It's hot and dry up here," Fofana said, "and cholera is a disease of warm moist areas."

"Don't be so sure of that," Renaud replied. The cholera vibrio is a fragile organism and heat kills it easily. But I've seen it survive in hot dry places."

Before we left the airport, Fofana said that he wanted to have a meeting in his office the following day about the cholera problem in Guinea and make plans for dealing with it if it spread to Mali.

"Since you're the epidemiologist here, Imperato," he said, "give us a brief rundown of the disease and its epidemiology. Make it succinct and easy for laymen to understand because I'm inviting the minister of the interior and the army chief of staff."

I gulped. What did I know about cholera, except what I read a short time before in my textbooks? I rushed home. It was eleven P.M. and the meeting was at ten A.M. It was like cramming for an exam in medical school.

The textbooks defined cholera as an acute contagious disease which caused vomiting, severe diarrhea and dehydration—loss of body water—all in a matter of hours. The diarrhea which leads to dehydration is due to the microbe and the poisonous toxins it produces. The microbe, first discovered by Koch, the renowned German bacteriologist, in 1883, looks like a comma under the microscope and is scientifically called *Vibrio cholerae*. The word cholera comes from the Greek word meaning "a flow of bile." The fatality rate from the disease ranges from 50 to 70 percent in untreated cases.

Cholera has probably been around in China and India since antiquity. From time to time it spread out of these areas to Europe and the Americas. In the nineteenth century there were five devastating worldwide epidemics, known as pandemics, and four reached the United States. In 1947 twenty thousand people died of cholera in the lower Nile valley where the disease had been absent for forty years. Over the years scientists learned that the microbe is transmitted from man to man through what is called the fecal-oral route. This means that feces containing the microbe get into the mouths of other people in some way. In India this happens in rivers where people defecate, urinate and drink the water at the same time. Someone with cholera defecating in the river spreads the microbe which is taken in by people drinking water nearby.

But in parts of the world with poor sanitation, the microbe can get onto foods, clothing and any number of objects which people touch. The greatest deterrent to cholera is good sanitation, clean water supplies, modern toilets with safe sewer systems and high levels of personal hygiene. Cholera could never get very far in the United States today or in most of Western Europe simply because of current sanitary habits. People don't regularly defecate in rivers or get their daily water supplies from them before they are thoroughly sanitized. The necessary links in the transmission chain just don't exist anymore. But they exist in places like Mali.

Scientists also discovered that there are three types of cholera microbes. They are the Ogawa, Inaba and El Tor variants. Dr. Renaud told us that the variant in Guinea was El Tor. It was first isolated in Egypt in 1905 at the El Tor quarantine station where pilgrims from Mecca were screened. El Tor cholera was widespread in the Middle East and in the Far East after 1905. In 1937 it caused a large epidemic in the Celebes and smoldered there until 1961. Then for reasons which aren't fully understood, El Tor moved out of the Celebes in June of that year. It invaded Java that month and by July was in Sarawak. In August it was in Macao and in September in Hong Kong and the Philippines. Everywhere it went it caused major epidemics. By 1965, El Tor was rolling westward into

Pakistan and Iraq. Two years later, in 1967, it moved across the Persian Gulf into the Arabian Peninsula. Then it crossed over into the Soviet Union in 1970.

That was as much as I could find out about it at the time. El Tor was causing the world's seventh known pandemic of cholera, one that had now reached Africa, not by contiguous land spread but by air. Somebody with cholera, probably a Guinean, flew into Conakry from the Soviet Union, traveled up into a rural area, became ill with the disease and then contaminated those around him. The unsanitary environment of rural Africa was ideal for this microbe which had never visited it before. It was completely at home.

It can take anywhere from a few hours to five days from the time someone swallows the cholera microbe until he comes down with the illness. Not everybody who takes in the microbe gets sick and some people have only mild illnesses. It's highly variable. There is a vaccine against cholera, but it gives protection to only 60 percent of the people who get it and that protection lasts for nine months at best. People have to receive two shots for the vaccine to give them maximum protection. This means that vaccination is not the ideal weapon for controlling cholera epidemics. Smallpox vaccine, by comparison, protects 95 percent of people for several years. So do many other vaccines.

The treatment of cholera sounds simple and it is. But it isn't available very often in remote rural areas where so many of the cases occur. People with cholera defecate water in huge quantities. They can lose up to twenty-five quarts of fluid in a matter of hours. Not only is the fluid lost, but also the body salts. Treatment then consists of intravenous infusions of salt solutions, enough to replace the quantity lost. Once this is done promptly, patients recover quickly. They stop vomiting, because the cause of the vomiting is an imbalance in their body salts. Intravenous salt solutions correct this. Antibiotics are then given by mouth to kill off the microbes still in the intestinal tract. It's easy to do this in any decent dispensary. But to do it in a remote corner of India or out in the wild rugged bush of Africa is a different story.

Once again I was a teacher only one step ahead of my pupils, explaining all this information at the meeting the next day. A lot of debate took place about the possibility of cholera coming into Mali from Guinea. In the end everyone agreed that we had to assume it would enter Mali sooner or later. But what should we do? Teach personal hygiene, build sewers, improve environmental sanitation? It all sounded great in a course in public health. But how were we going to achieve it in a country as big as Mali with millions of people spread out over a rural wilderness?

"I've decided to take some immediate steps," Fofana said. "All plane flights between Bamako and Conakry are to be suspended; all river travel on the Niger between our two countries is to be stopped immediately. No foods may be imported into Mali from Guinea. All travelers coming into Mali from Guinea overland are to be put into frontier quarantine stations for five days. Anyone who's been to Guinea in the previous five days and arrives here by air is to be quarantined until the five days are up."

Sougoule suggested Mali set up a *cordon sanitaire*—a health barrier along the frontier with Guinea. "Cholera won't get past that barrier. That I guarantee," he said, shaking his head with determined emphasis.

No one believed him. The frontier of several hundred miles ran through sparsely inhabited rural areas and wilderness. People crossed back and forth over it at will. But Sougoule was persistent in demanding that he as head of the Hygiene Service be authorized to set up his medical Maginot Line.

"A good suggestion," Fofana said, half hiding a smile. "You can use your sanitary inspectors along the main road and tracks." It was a chance to get Sougoule out of the way to where he could do little damage.

"I plan to vaccinate all of the villages one mile in from the frontier," Sougoule said, "and I'm going to hold all travelers coming out of Guinea in quarantine posts at the frontier for five days."

We all listened attentively, but smiled inside. Cholera could easily get carried past Sougoule's frontier posts and vaccinated villages. His was an effort without much promise.

Fofana made an appeal to the World Health Organization for cholera vaccine. The organization had been designated by the cholera-vaccine manufacturing countries as the distributor. Supplies were limited and had to be carefully distributed. Mali eventually got close to half a million doses. Fofana also sent out appeals for intravenous fluids and asked the American embassy for assistance in supplying them.

At the lazaret, and out in the cholera treatment centers, special cholera cots were made in large numbers. They were made of impermeable rubber with large holes in the center through which the watery feces of patients would pass through a sealed tube into a bucket containing disinfectant.

It amazed me that the Malians got all of this into place in three weeks—the IV fluids, the vaccine, the cholera treatment stations and the cots. In addition, the health education section of the Ministry of Health gave daily advisories over Radio Mali on how to prevent cholera. The Malians running health affairs in the country were both well trained and experienced in dealing with major epidemics. All of them had been through the meningitis epidemic and the yellow fever epidemic which followed it.

Once all these preparations were in place, we stopped and waited. A week went by and no cases were reported from adjacent countries. Then in late September, almost a month after Dr. Renaud's stopover visit in Bamako, Sierra Leone announced that it had cholera. And from there seagoing fishermen carried it over to neighboring Liberia in a matter of days. It moved eastward through Liberia and finally reached the capital, Monrovia, the first week of October. I flew down to Monrovia to appraise the situation. The disease was limited to a shantytown of fishermen, but within a few days spread like wildfire through the whole city. I telegraphed my findings to Bamako.

The disease kept moving, at an intensified tempo. By October 17 it was in Abidjan, the capital of the Ivory Coast. A number of merchants had brought it into the Ivory Coast from Liberia. One of them died in Abidjan and was buried in his home village a hundred miles to the north. As friends and relatives carried his body north, they stopped in villages along the way where ceremonies were held over the remains. Five days after the body passed through, cholera broke out in the villages.

Some of the optimists in Bamako argued that the disease would spare the dry savannah.

"Look," one of them said at the weekly strategy meeting, "it has only hit the coast—Sierra Leone, Liberia, Ivory Coast, Ghana and yesterday Togo. It's the twelfth of November already. If it were coming north, it would have by now."

"He's right," Sougoule said, just in from a few days down on

131

the Guinea frontier. "Two and a half months and nothing north of the rain forest."

Cholera had pretty much stuck to the coast. Day by day it edged its way forward, a dozen miles here, fifty miles there. It wasn't skipping over areas, leaping ahead hundreds of miles and suddenly breaking out in a far-off place. If it was coming to Mali, it would edge its way in from either Guinea or the Ivory Coast.

What puzzled me was why it hadn't crossed the Guinea border already and spilled into Mali, especially since the disease supposedly started close by. Sougoule had done a pretty good job of policing the main road and some of the tracks. But there were hundreds of miles of bush beyond his control. Surely if cholera were on the other side it would have come over by now. I didn't know what to make of it. Neither did anyone else. Sougoule didn't have any doubts though. As far as he was concerned, his Maginot Line was working. He had set up similar procedures along the Ivory Coast border. Everyone coming across had to have a valid cholera vaccination certificate. Otherwise they were held in a quarantine camp for five days.

A week later, November 19, the first cool-air masses of the winter season moved over Bamako. They lowered the midday temperatures into the seventies, from their usual level 40 degrees higher. This was the most comfortable season in Mali, but it never lasted very long. By February the temperatures soared up again over a hundred.

My phone rang around four-fifteen P.M.

"Hallo," I said.

"Hallo, Docteur Imperato?"

"Oui," I answered.

"C'est le Ministre qui vous appelle. Attendez un moment."

I waited. When Fofana got on the line he said in a grave voice, "Le cholera nous a frappé à Mopti."

"Mopti!" I exclaimed. "How can that be? It's over fifteen hundred miles from the nearest cholera outbreak on the coast."

"I know," Fofana said. "But that's where it's hit us."

"When did it happen?"

"About an hour ago. Dr. Diallo sent a radio message from the governor's office. He said there are seven cases among merchants from the Ivory Coast."

132

"The Ivory Coast? How did they get through?"

"They snuck through the quarantine controls at the border on a bush track and drove right up to Mopti from Abidjan."

"What's happening now?"

"Can't say for sure. I don't have any further information. Diallo knows what to do. I'm sure he's already put things into motion."

"Are you going up?"

"No. I'm sending Keita. It's best we stay here for the time being. This is just the start. There is no way of knowing what will happen now."

I put the phone down. I was stunned. Cholera in Mopti. Incredible! I knew now that we had a disaster on our hands.

Mopti is a town of fifty thousand people, built of mud brick on three islands in the middle of the largest swamp in West Africa, the great Inland Delta of the Niger. The delta is the size of the state of Maine. The town is the crossroads of the middle Niger, the major trading center between Bamako and Timbuktu to the north. Commerce is the very life of Mopti and its existence is animated by its markets which attract traders from hundreds of miles around, from Mauritania, Senegal, Nigeria, Ghana, Ivory Coast and even from Morocco. The stalls are full of heaps of spices, salt from the Sahara, leather goods and saddles, beautifully painted pottery, firearms, piles of Maria Theresa dollars, cotton, wool, cloth, foodstuffs of every sort, dried fish and heaps of beautifully woven blankets.

Although Mopti is picturesque, it is also drastically crude and unhealthful, a city where contagious diseases like typhoid fever and malaria are present all the time. The water table beneath the islands is so high that latrines can't be dug. So they are built in one of the rooms on the ground floor of houses with the toilets above on the second floor. Seepage occurs and often the walls of the latrines break, spilling their accumulated contents into the gutters. People in Mopti get their water from wells and from the Bani River which flows into the Niger just in front of the town. The Bani River comes close to being a sewer at Mopti. Several bacteriologic surveys had been done. They all came up with the same results. The river was a cesspool, full of every imaginable microbe.

November 19 was a Thursday. That's the day of Mopti's weekly fair. Almost ten thousand people come into Mopti on market day, on donkeys, on foot, on horses, on camels and in canoes which sail up and down the Niger from neighboring villages. Scores of trucks and buses roll in over the road that runs on top of the nine-mile-long dike connecting Mopti to the mainland. Itinerant merchants from all over West Africa show up in Mopti on market day. They and the tens of thousands of other people use the Bani River to wash and to drink in . . . and its waters as a toilet. Sanitary conditions were at their worst in Mopti on market day and on that day the Bani River was a visible sewer.

What was different about this market day was the presence of the cholera vibrio in the waters of the Bani for the first time in history. No one could see it. But it was there.

Late in the afternoon, a merchant from the Ivory Coast was carried to the hospital suffering from vomiting, diarrhea and severe dehydration. Ten minutes later, six of his companions were carried in with the same illness.

Dr. Diallo, the chief medical officer, took one look at them and knew it was cholera. He had the men taken to the lazaret where they were hooked up to intravenous infusions. And then he tried to call Fofana in Bamako. The telephone lines were out. He raced to the governor's office, told him what happened and sent a radio message to Fofana. There was a lot of static and they could hardly hear one another. But Diallo was able to get the essential points over to Fofana.

Diallo imposed an immediate quarantine on the town. No one was to leave and no one was to enter. But the afternoon had worn on already and thousands had left. The big canoes loaded with people and merchandise were on their way down river, sailing toward scores of villages around Lake Debo and along the numerous creeks which led to Timbuktu. Soldiers from the Mopti garrison blocked the road leading out of town. But they couldn't stop the hundreds of people who fled in canoes. Under the cover of darkness, the canoes slithered by them in the high grass, along the lagoons and canals. And so did the cholera vibrio.

134

CHAPTER 11

DEATH ALONG THE RIVER

The Niger River was in flood, a wide brown muddy torrent, rushing on its way to the sea. Downstream from Mopti it flowed through the great lakes of the Inland Delta and then on to Timbuktu and beyond the Niger Bend. Above Mopti, the rains had turned the plains of central Mali into a immense swamp, a world of blues and greens and maritime infinity. The sun rose here between the reeds as a giant red disc and set behind a trail of changing light—red, orange, gold and silver, painting the surface of the waters with whimsical creative hues. In this part of Mali, I always felt I was sailing on the sea. I sensed no limits and heard the sounds of water moving upon itself, going nowhere in particular, but constantly on the move. Sky and water all around is what I saw and there was always a fresh breeze, gently moving through the tall stands of swamp grass, dancing on the water and lifting flocks of water fowl high above my head in gentle lazy circles.

But unlike the sea, this was not an immensity lacking a permanent human presence. For scattered across these flood plains were island villages, hidden in the grass, where life had gone on for centuries cut off from the outside world by water and swamp, by custom and time. Man's life depended on the river, on its rising and falling, on the migration of fish attuned to the currents, on the

135

grasses which sprouted after the flood, which fed the cattle, goats and sheep. Man had long ago put himself in synchrony with this river and shaped his life around its cycles.

When the waters on the plains receded, the herdsmen moved down from the high plateaus and grazed their herds on the verdant lawn left behind by the river. They stayed there, close to the reeds, until the rains fell again, and then they moved back waiting for the river to regenerate the earth. The fishermen had their cycles too, moving downstream with the falling crest, on toward Lake Debo and the other lakes which spread out toward the eastern skies. Below their canoes moved millions of fish, following an ancient instinct, poorly understood by man, but well observed. Then when the rains began, the fishermen returned upstream again, following the fish and finally settled into their island villages, unable to reach their prey, now protected by dark depths and fearsome currents. They were all there now, on those islands, surrounded by water and swamp, which for generations had given life.

The Niger was the river of life. But soon it would become a river of death. For its currents now carried what was unknown to all, to the minstrels and holy men, to the chiefs and elders. All their collective wisdom and all their reserves of ancient oral tradition would fail them when faced with this unseen enemy. It was sailing toward them, up the narrow creeks and across the quiet marshes, finding its way into their wells and drinking cups. It would contaminate their hands and feet, their faces and their clothing. It would follow them into their homes and into their mosques, to the very altars where they worshiped their ancestors. It would strike down the rich and the poor, the old and the young, and leave a permanent mark on the memory of this land.

Alfa Diallo sailed out of Mopti in a large canoe late in the afternoon. The canoe carried him downstream, toward Akka, his home village which lay two days ahead, beyond Lake Debo. He was a cloth merchant who had come to the Mopti fair a few days before with his ten-year-old son Moussa. The Mopti fair was a busy place in November; the crops were in and people started traveling up and down the river to trade, visit and discuss. The season of isolation ended in November and movement was intense, a response to months of retreat and isolation. Alfa had done a brisk business in Mopti and sailed home with bales of spices, mangoes, mirrors and combs which he had bought with some of his profits

It was early in the afternoon when he and Moussa left their stall in the crowded market to go down to the river to wash and drink. Leaving their goods in the care of a kinsman, they made their way through the jostling jungle of hawkers and buyers. There was a refreshing breeze along the river and air that was clear of the heaviness which hung in the market. They folded their clothes in a neat pile on the shore and waded into the stream. There was no shame to nakedness under these skies and up and down the bank men and women moved in and out of the water with that comfort only innocence can bestow. The river was full of people, traders from Bamako and Timbuktu, from Upper Volta and Ghana and from the Ivory Coast. It was a place to relax, to drink and wash, to meet and chat and get away from the heat of the sun.

Alfa and Moussa came out of the water. "That was good, wasn't it?" Alfa said to his son.

"Yes it was. But when are we going home?"

"In a little while."

"You said that before."

"I know, but it won't be long now." Alfa put on his robe. "I have to get the goods loaded into the canoe for Akka." He patted Moussa on the head.

Alfa went back to his stall. The afternoon had worn on and people had begun packing up their goods. Some left in large trucks, traveling on top of mounds of baggage, their heads wrapped up in scarves as protection against the evening air. Others could afford more luxurious accommodations in minibuses or tarpaulin-covered Peugeot pickup trucks and the aristocrats of the land-traveling merchants exited in Peugeot station wagons. But the real life of this market came and went on the river, in large canoes over a hundred feet long, covered with straw canopies. Some had tall masts standing on the stern from which huge, supple rectangular pieces of cloth fluttered like the medieval arms of some great prince. These canoes were created from skills which descended the centuries through numerous generations. But now many of them had inboard motors and had discarded the rows of oarsmen whose muscle power once took them as far east as Timbuktu.

It took a couple of hours for Alfa to wind up his affairs and get a group of porters to carry his bales down to the *Amadou*, the canoe that would take them home. Once on board, they had to wait another hour for other merchants to board and arrange their heavy baggage around the boat to the satisfaction of the captain. And then as the evening chill began to rise up from the water, they set sail. The canoe puttered out of the little cover and into the main channel where the swift current negated any use of its motor. Downstream they went with incredible speed, past the imposing edifice that was the governor's residence and the cream-colored buildings which Alfa explained were the hospital and dispensary. Villages and people flashed by on the bank for a while, and then as the sun set, they moved slowly into a world of cool stillness where only the shrieks of water fowl broke the great silence.

The canoe stopped at the village of Sendigue for the night, and passengers found lodging wherever they could. Toward midnight some traders arrived in a small canoe from Mopti. Alfa heard a loud commotion and got up from his mat to see what was happening.

"A great curse appeared in Mopti," one of them said excitedly. "The soldiers wouldn't let anyone leave. But we were able to get out after dark."

"What is this curse?" Alfa asked.

"It is a curse on all traders for not paying their taxes."

"For not paying their taxes?"

"Yes, only traders are cursed."

"Who has cursed them?"

"The government agents have paid some evil *imams* to do this, to put fear into us so that we will pay our taxes in the future. We are no fools; we weren't going to be held captive in Mopti so that the curse could fall on us."

"Did you see anyone with this curse?"

"No," the trader replied. "But others did and they said that those with the curse pass their urine from their rectum and from their mouth. It flows out of them like the river, never stopping until they die."

"This is a strange curse," Alfa said somewhat incredulously. He didn't know what to make of it. No news of it had reached him when he was in Mopti.

"You got out before they blocked the port and the road," the trader told him.

Alfa left the traders and the crowd of chattering villagers and went back to the hut where he had been sleeping with Moussa.

"What is it?" Moussa asked.

"Nothing. Just some ignorant men babbling a silly story about a curse."

None of the others in Sendigue shared Alfa's view that the traders were babbling. Miracles, curses and magic were daily occurrences in the lives of these people. They had no reason to doubt what the traders said. They willingly believed. Yet for men like Alfa who had been to school for a few years, belief wasn't so easily given.

True, he thought the soldiers may have been stopping people from leaving. But they have done that before, to check licenses and identification cards. That's what must have been going on. And with those thoughts Alfa went to sleep.

Seven hundred miles away, I too went to sleep, but with the knowledge that a great disaster was in the making. An uneasy calm always fills the time between the first appearance of a disease and the subsequent epidemic. Medical detectives know that this calm represents the incubation period of the disease—the time it takes from the microbe's first entry into the body until the victim shows symptoms and signs of the disease. I wondered how many people were incubating cholera, where they had gone to and how quickly they would pass it on to those around them.

My sleep wasn't sound. I tossed around in bed, woke up and thought. I knew for certain that the cholera vibrio was alive in their intestines. They would feel perfectly well for about five days, the time it takes for the microbe to produce enough toxin to make them sick. And then it would strike them, not in gradual warning stages like the flu, but like a bolt of lightning cutting its way down a perfectly blue sky.

Downstream in Sendigue, Alfa and his son slept soundly. A strong silence reigned outside. The doves and crickets had long since stopped singing and only the sound of the river hurrying on its way drifted across the plains, losing its identity in the rustling of the cool breeze.

I thought about the cholera toxin and how lethal it was to the lining of the intestines. It caused the intestines to pour out all of the body's fluids. Once it began taking effect those fluids came out like a torrent, turning the victim into a dried-up prune. The body salts flowed out too, depriving the heart of the proper balance it needs to

139

continue beating. Eventually the heart stops beating. Someone perfectly well at ten in the morning is suddenly shriveled up and dead by two in the afternoon!

The *Amadou* set sail for Lake Debo at sunrise, somewhat earlier than usual because the captain and some of the passengers wanted to get as far away as possible from Mopti and its curse. Alfa looked ahead over the high prow of the vessel and saw the open blue waters of Debo, the "Lake of the Woman." That great lake held within it a reservoir of mythological beliefs and spiritual powers. For the Peul nomads believe that Tyanaba, a supernatural ancestor and the first herdsman, lives in the depths of Debo with his wife. It was she who brought him there and who gives magic to the waters. At the bottom of the lake are Tyanaba's supernatural herds. They come up out of the water at night and graze on the shores. For this reason, the Peul take their cattle to Debo as the dry season ends, so that they can drink the waters and come into contact with their own supernatural ancestors.

"Debo will stop the curse," the captain said to Alfa. "It will never pass her."

"There is no curse," Alfa replied, "just the talk of men who have tongues like women. It is all nonsense."

"It is not nonsense," the captain insisted. "Several others came to Sendigue last night. They say the same thing. It must be true."

As the *Amadou* entered Lake Debo, a meeting took place at the Ministry of Health. Fofana said that he had sent out orders over the radio telephone system operated by the Ministry of the Interior. All of the riverine villages within a hundred kilometers of Mopti were to be vaccinated.

"I know," he said, anticipating my question, "that many of those villages are isolated because of the flood and that the vaccination teams may not get there in time. But we have to do something."

It was a gamble. The cholera vibrio already had a day's start. Four more days and all hell would break loose, long before vaccination teams could reach those villages.

"Even if people are vaccinated," I said, "it will take a week for them to develop protection against cholera. And the vaccine isn't all that good anyway."

140

"It's a terrible predicament," Fofana said, "but we have to try it for whatever good it does."

"What do we do about Bamako?" a representative from the Ministry of Interior asked.

"Imperato, what do we do?" Fofana asked. "Do we vaccinate now, or wait? You tell us."

"We wait, until the last possible moment. Then we vaccinate."

"When will that be?" Fofana asked.

"I don't know yet, but once the epidemic starts, I'll be able to tell you within a couple of days. I have to see how fast it moves upstream. And I don't know yet if it will come in along the road."

Later that day, Fofana announced over Radio Mali that cholera had broken out in Mopti. Health educators from the ministry got on the air and explained what cholera was, how it could be treated and how it could be prevented.

"Boil your drinking water," they urged, "and the ablution waters used at the mosque."

The *Amadou* moved through Lake Debo, cut off from the world and from what was going on upstream. There were no radios on board so the continuous health-education lectures in all the national languages didn't reach the ship. But up and down the river and across Mali, wherever there were transistor radios, the word spread that the Apollo disease—the Africans' name for cholera—was in Mopti.

I felt tremendously frustrated not being able to combat this scourge because I didn't know where it was, where it was going and what it would ultimately do. I could only take comfort in the fact that Fofana had wisely set up cholera treatment centers all over the country and that I had poised vaccination teams with jet injectors and vaccine up and down the river.

The *Amadou* docked at the village of Guidio Saree late in the afternoon. And it was there that Alfa learned what had happened in Mopti.

"Cholera?" he asked himself. He had never heard of it. Neither had the captain nor anyone else. But from what the speaker was saying over the radio it was the same disease the traders had described the night before.

That afternoon, Fofana received some details on the outbreak in

Mopti and called me. "The traders went into the river to defecate," he said.

"Where along the river?"

"Near the port."

"Oh, my God! That means they were upstream from everyone else who went into the river. All those people who bathed and drank along the shore must have come into contact with the vibrio."

"Let's hope the water diluted the concentration of the organism," Fofana said.

"If it did, then the disease won't be so bad in those incubating it right now." I was grasping at straws, hoping for the best, when clearly the worst was going to happen. But the possibility was real that only mild cases would develop in people who had swallowed small numbers of microbes.

The *Amadou* docked in Akka on the twenty-second of November. Hawa Diallo and her three other sons came down to the river's edge to meet her husband and Moussa. There was a joyful reunion. She had heard about the Apollo disease, the illness which the people of Akka said was sent down from the sky by the Americans from invisible ships which they sailed up there. Alfa shook his head. In Mopti it was the government which caused it and now in Akka the Americans. What he didn't know was that in Timbuktu it would be the French, in Gao the Russians and in Kangaba the Guineans. Wild though these rumors may have been, they were man's attempt to assign causality to the unknown and in so doing enable himself to deal with it. Cholera didn't fit into the known spectrum of diseases. It had to be probed and discovered, opened and laid bare and made subject to the powers of herbs and healers, incantations and talismans. The *imams* readied themselves, some confident that they could defeat this new disease. They were mistaken. For this disease wasn't a fever which lingered for days and provided time for readings from the Koran. It came and went in a flash, struck and killed before the book could even be opened and the verse chosen. They would learn about cholera and how it killed, and once they did they would recoil and retreat as never before, admitting defeat within their hearts but not beyond. They would say it was God and that "inshalla—God willing" it would pass and leave this land. And before His will men were without power. They

142

had to suffer and obey and submit to His will and pray for forgiveness for whatever it was they had done to deserve this travail.

The disasters of Africa are often announced without fear, for their natures are known as well as the ancient means for dealing with them. But the nature of cholera wasn't known, and when it struck, panic and fear spread all over the country, like an epidemic itself, clearing a path for what was to follow. Alfa and his wife worried. Two days had gone by and the radio spoke of nothing else but this strange new disease. The chief had assembled all of the people the night before to tell them that the dispensary had special water in plastic bags sent from Bamako. Once the disease struck, this water had to be put into a victim's blood with a needle. The nurse knew how to do this; he had been to Mopti two weeks before to learn. But the *imam* of Akka said that the disease wouldn't touch the village. "I have protected you all in the past, have I not?" he asked, interrupting the chief. A murmur of assent came back from the crowd.

Alfa was a devout Moslem, but he had little confidence in the healing powers of the *imam*. His charms and incantations are worthless, Alfa thought. He remembered the Kodak film cartridge filled with a red bead and a scrap of paper with scribblings from the Koran which the *imam* had given to his sister when she couldn't become pregnant. It cost ten thousand francs! That was twenty dollars, the monthly wage of a civil servant in Bamako, as much cash as a herdsman would see in a year.

"We must do what the radio says," Alfa said, rising to his feet. "The government doctors know this disease and we do not. You have never seen it," he said to the *imam.*

"I have seen it," the *imam* retorted with an eloquent lie. "Allah has shown it to me in a dream and He will guide me in protecting you. Those who defy Allah's will invite their own death."

The chief and the nurse kept silent. They feared the *imam.* "You, Alfa Diallo, son of Isaac Diallo, pray at the mosque, but you are a nonbeliever. God is displeased with you."

"You speak wrongly, holy man," retorted Alfa. "I do not believe in your magic, nor does Allah, and you know it in your heart."

"Blasphemy! Insolence! May Allah curse you and all your house with this disease, Alfa Diallo. You will pay for your disbelief."

143

* * *

Flocks of white egrets flew over Akka in the cool of the morning air, standing out in sharp contrast to the blue of the sky. They flew eastward toward Lake Niangaye and Lake Haribongo, etching a white streak toward the distant horizon. Fishermen drew in their nets along Lake Debo and their basket traps from their moorings on the banks of the Issa Ber and the Bara Issa. Alfa went down to his stall in the market, to sell the produce he had brought downstream from Mopti. It was a sleepy place, of quiet conversation and pleasant thoughts. No hurried pace stepped into this place, even on the day of the weekly fair. Urgency and commotion were aliens in the passive gaze of the old men who sat and prayed. They prayed for what had been and for what might have been, forgiveness for the past and reward in the eternal ahead.

Alfa felt his stomach rumble. He brushed it aside. He had experienced this many times before. But as the minutes passed by, he felt strange. It was as if suddenly all his internal being were going to gush out. He sat down and wiped his brow. His mouth began to feel wet with that unsettling salivation that heralds something worse to come. And then it came, in great heaves, pouring out onto the dry ground and disappearing beneath a darkened spot of earth. The old men were jolted. They came over. He couldn't hold it in. The water poured out of his rectum, soiling his robe and cascading down into the earth. They called some young men and had Alfa carried to the dispensary and then one of them went to tell his wife. Alfa felt his life flowing out of him. It disappeared into the earth in a trail of dampened dust all the way to the dispensary.

So this was it, he thought, the dreaded cholera. Within minutes he couldn't think anymore.

Hawa came running to the dispensary with Moussa. She shrieked when she saw her husband. The water came out of him, from his mouth and rectum, belching waves of clear fluid, sent out with moans and panting. The nurse told her to wait outside. He inserted the intravenous and opened it wide. The fluid dripped in but he was frightened because for every few drops that went in a liter came out.

Up in Bamako it was a warm day, the day I knew we would hear news of other cases of cholera. Fofana called me around noon. "Cholera has broken out in Diafarabe!" he exclaimed.

144

"Diafarabe? That's a hundred miles from Mopti."

"Yes I know," he said, "and worse, it's in Goundam, two hundred miles downstream."

"Unbelievable! This disease has moved three hundred miles in five days. Why, down on the coast it took a month to get that far."

"We have to plan on its moving with speed from now on," Fofana said. "Before we know it Bamako will be in jeopardy."

The only good news Fofana had was that Mopti's population of sixty thousand had been vaccinated and that people there were boiling their water. But he couldn't say what was going on in the rural villages. I could imagine, though. If cholera were in Diafarabe and in Goundam, it was everywhere else in between. Akka was a hundred miles upstream from Goundam. Although I didn't know it at the time, cholera had broken out there among most of those who had traveled from Mopti on the *Amadou*.

The nurse decided to hook up a second bottle in Alfa's arm. One just couldn't keep pace with what was pouring out of him. An old man who had been in the marketplace said that the captain of the *Amadou* had just come down with the same sickness. His family had taken him to the *imam*, who was reading passages from the Koran over him.

Two hours went by and then the vomiting and diarrhea stopped. The intravenous fluid dripped into Alfa's veins, and gradually the wrinkles in his skin disappeared, his cheeks filled out and his eyes came to life. By evening he recovered. But the captain was dead. His body poured out into the earth in streams of water as the *imam* prayed over him.

Others who were on the *Amadou* fell ill, but they came to the dispensary and abandoned the *imam*. Word spread that Alfa lived and that the captain was dead. "And Moussa?" Alfa asked his wife as he got up from the mat in the dispensary late in the evening and prepared to go home.

"He is fine," she said. "The illness did not touch him."

Moussa, like others who were exposed, didn't develop the disease, probably because he didn't swallow a large number of microbes. Or he may not have swallowed any at all as he bathed and drank in the river that day.

Downstream from Mopti, cholera caused the worst disaster anyone could remember. It spread like wildfire, carrying off half the populations of isolated villages. Sarafere's population of 828 was reduced to 426. But in areas like Akka where there were cholera treatment facilities, the mortality was less than 5 percent. In Mopti, where medical facilities were pretty sophisticated, there were only two hundred cases and fourteen deaths. "That's a near miracle!" I said to Fofana.

"I agree," he said, "but they did boil their water and cases were treated right away."

The disease kept moving. By December 4, fifteen days after it appeared in Mopti, it broke out in Koulikoro, five hundred miles upstream and only thirty miles from Bamako.

The speed of this thing is unbelievable! I thought. It didn't do this down in Liberia and the Ivory Coast.

Fofana and I went up to Koulikoro. It's a riverine town of two thousand and the railhead for the trains which go down to Dakar on the coast. People travel between Bamako and Koulikoro every day on the train. The river isn't navigable because of a series of rapids. We hadn't been there more than an hour when Fofana decided to block the road and the railroad and quarantine the town. Not that this would do much good. Cholera was rolling up toward Bamako, the largest city in Mali, with two hundred thousand susceptible people living in squalid unhygienic conditions. We called the ministry and Fofana gave the go-ahead to vaccinate the city.

We then went to the lazaret in Koulikoro, set up in an old warehouse. There were fifteen people there with cholera. The nurses in charge had misunderstood instructions. Instead of giving as much intravenous solution as was needed, they gave one liter and then stopped. Fofana was angry.

"Put those intravenouses back!" he ordered. "And keep them going until the patients stop vomiting and passing water."

One three-year-old girl was in extremis—a medical term meaning at death's door. She had been brought in several hours earlier, soon enough to have saved her life. But the nurses had given her one liter of fluid and had called it quits. She continued to vomit and pass half her body fluids over the next few hours. I put an intravenous into her femoral vein. It is a large deep vein in the groin. It was our only hope since all her other veins had collapsed and were nonfunctioning. The intravenous started flowing. I looked up and

146

watched the fluid dripping down into the plastic tubing. I felt relieved. She would be saved. But I was wrong. No sooner had the life-giving fluid begun to flow than she stopped breathing.

"She could have been saved," I muttered to Fofana.

"I know," he said in a downcast tone, "had we come an hour earlier."

Out in the back of the lazaret, a young man was stretched out on the ground. His left arm twitched back and forth.

"He's been dead for several hours," the chief nurse said.

"But his arm is moving."

"Doesn't matter. That's part of dying."

I couldn't believe what I was seeing and hearing. True, the man was dried up like a prune and wasn't breathing. And I couldn't get a pulse or a heartbeat. But the twitching in his arm told me that he hadn't died more than a few moments before. Involuntary muscle movements like this aren't unusual in people dying of cholera. But I was certain that the man had had a heartbeat and a pulse an hour before, several hours after the nurses had given him up for dead. I had reason to doubt their story and so did Fofana. He made a call to Bamako and asked that two nurses be sent out immediately to take over the supervision of the lazaret.

The chief nurse wasn't mean or unfeeling, just ignorant.

"If he's been dead for so long then why hasn't he been buried?" I asked.

"No one knows him. He's an itinerant worker from up north who lived with two other friends. They died yesterday."

"You mean there's no one in this town who'll bury him?"

"Why should they? He's not their relative!"

I wasn't shocked by the nurse's reply because I knew that getting a decent burial wasn't a right. It was a privilege. In Bamako, strangers without kin and nonconforming Moslems were buried by prisoners, unless someone else was willing to do it. The prisoners shouted obscenities at the corpse as they took it to the cemetery and continued this as they dug the grave, lowered the body and filled in the earth.

Fofana ordered the nurse to get some of the soldiers from the local garrison to bury the dead man. It would be a more dignified burial than one carried out by prisoners.

147

"But how will his family know he's dead?" I asked Fofana.

"They won't," he said sadly. "A few years will pass by and when he doesn't return they will assume he died."

He saw my reaction. "Life is cruel in Africa, isn't it?"

The next day, the vaccinators continued to vaccinate Bamako's population. Within two days, they gave 234,610 shots. The disease hadn't moved out of Koulikoro and the only cases there that day were among the old men who buried the dead. These old Moslems didn't believe in vaccinations. Five days after they washed and buried their kin, they came down with cholera. As I was to learn several weeks later, the *imam* in Akka also contracted the disease in the course of treating people and he died along with them.

In Segou, a town of forty thousand downstream from Bamako, one of the town's leading *imams* claimed he could prevent cholera. People flocked to him and for a fee equal to twenty American dollars—a month's wage in Mali—he wrote verses from the Koran on their backs with a BIC ballpoint pen. Thinking they were protected, people didn't boil their water or come out to be vaccinated. And when they developed cholera they went to see him. He treated them with more ballpoint inscriptions and most of them died. The chief medical officer began to suspect something when he noticed that most of the deaths from the disease were coming from one section of the town. He went there and started talking to people and to some of the victims who were brought to the lazaret. It was then that he uncovered what the *imam* was doing. He notified the police and they arrested the *imam*. The medical officer was perplexed that the *imam* hadn't contracted cholera himself. He discovered why. The *imam* had been vaccinated three times!

We held our breaths and waited. Would the vaccinations protect Bamako? Experts said that vaccination wasn't an effective preventive measure. Fofana had received that advice from the World Health Organization and I had gotten it from CDC. But the British textbooks of tropical medicine said the contrary. It worked, they claimed, provided most of the population were vaccinated. That we had done. And I hoped that the British with all their experience in India were right.

Within a few days we had an answer. Cholera swung around to the north of Bamako, sparing the city, and then came back down to the river again upstream.

148

"The British were right!" I shouted to Jean Duval over the phone after cholera had passed Bamako.

"Of course they're right," he said. "They always are. Didn't you know that?"

There were few villages along the Niger upstream from Bamako. The area was a dense wooded wilderness, especially near the Guinea border. Without people there, cholera wouldn't appear. But outside of Bamako the disease came into contact with the railway. It abandoned the river and started traveling westward, hitting towns and villages along the tracks. Then at Bafoulabe, where the tracks cross the headwaters of the Senegal River, the disease moved onto the river. It went down the Senegal River and the railway a thousand miles to the sea, carried by travelers, merchants and fishermen.

By the end of December over four thousand cases of cholera were reported in Mali and a thousand deaths. That number was a gross underestimate. In hundreds of rural villages no one knew how many cases there were and how many died. It moved out of the country as quickly as it had come, down the Niger into the Niger Republic and down the tracks and Senegal River into Senegal. But it remained behind in scattered places, causing a few cases at a time. Cholera was permanently implanted in West Africa, not as a raging pandemic, but as a smoldering permanent disease, causing a few cases here and there every year. No one can say when the next epidemic will come. But everyone knows that it will.

CHAPTER 12

HOME AGAIN

At the end of 1971 I had been in Mali for five years. Smallpox was eradicated, measles controlled and Mali's health services strengthened. Gradually the feeling came over me that I should return home. I had accomplished what I had been sent out to do and felt fulfilled. I had learned a great deal during these years and had grown from a neophyte trainee to an experienced medical detective. This maturation process had been greatly influenced by some of my older Malian colleagues. Even though I had been sent out to help them, very often it was they who showed me the way. I had seen almost every imaginable tropical disease found in Africa, had learned to diagnose and treat them and I saw them in the larger social and economic contexts in which they existed.

Uprooting myself from Africa was a major decision, a traumatic move, but one that I knew was in my best interests. I had been out of the mainstream of American medicine for five years. Technology in diagnosis and treatment had leaped forward and left me and my knowledge and skills far behind. True, I had faithfully read the leading medical journals which made their way over to me by sea. But reading was one thing; seeing and experiencing were another. I was aware that if I stayed any longer I would become rusty and have a difficult time catching up.

Fofana and some of my other Malian colleagues tried to persuade me to remain. I was flattered, but I knew that I had to return home. Even Sougoule stood drawn and sad as I moved my personal effects out of the office. "I will never forget you," he said. "You did a lot for Mali."

Sougoule had provided me with an important life experience. Men are complex, with good and bad all rolled into one. As trite as this sounds, it was something I didn't fully understand when I arrived in Mali. I saw everything in absolute terms. There was no middle ground, no gray zone. I had laughed at Sougoule's medical Maginot Line. But it worked. The presence of his inspectors along the border served as a psychologic deterrent to a population keenly sensitized to repression. That was something I hadn't foreseen, something not covered in any medical textbook.

I gradually came to terms with leaving Mali, so that when the day of my departure arrived I felt a great inner calm. It was a very cool morning, I remember, scented with mango blossoms and the fruit of kapok trees. I had first arrived in Mali during this season and my mind flashed back to those early days. I got up to pack a few last things before the sun rose above the Manding Hills. The house was empty now except for the furniture. All of my belongings had been crated and sent off by truck to Abidjan in the Ivory Coast, where they would be put on a ship bound for New York.

I opened the front door to let in the breeze from the garden. But when I did, I found my staff gathered beneath the trees. My plane wasn't due to leave for another three hours. And yet there they were! I asked them why they had come so early, but they couldn't give me a reply. This didn't mean they didn't have a reason. I knew them too well for that. They looked mournful and sad, adrift on the waters of an uncertain future. Their lives had been intertwined with mine and with our work in Mali for so long and now all was being unraveled. It was they who guided me through the bush, across the plains and over the mountains, who assisted me when I fought smallpox, meningitis and cholera. They always walked in the lead, cautioning me where to step, and now they looked to me to show them a safe path into the future.

Before leaving Mali, I had read a great deal about what psychiatrists call "reentry shock." It had been extensively studied among returning Peace Corps volunteers. The reverse had also been studied. It's called "culture shock," the accumulated feelings which result when someone enters an alien society. Reentry shock is similar. Absence abroad makes someone's home appear alien when he returns to it after a long time. Under normal circumstances, New York would have appeared alien to me after my years in Mali. But it was all the more so because of the convulsing social revolution which had taken place in the United States in the late 1960s.

In medicine it wasn't only drugs and diagnostic technology that had drastically changed, but many other things as well. Medicaid and Medicare had been implemented since my departure. I didn't know what they were. They could have been ice-cream mixes for all I knew. Little did I know then that in five years I would be Commissioner of Health of New York City with major responsibilities for the Medicaid program. American medical-school graduates were leaving New York City by the droves, going out to California and to the eastern slopes of the Rockies. Internships and residencies which had once been hard to get in hospitals in Brooklyn now went begging. Hospitals had to fill them with foreign medical graduates. Young American doctors were no longer opening private practices in many areas of the city. They said that neighborhoods had shifted, crime was high and the quality of life poor.

I wasn't sure yet if I wanted to continue working as an epidemiologist and so I decided to explore a number of other possibilities. I followed up a lead on a position in a large medical center. The director of the medical service was a specialist in infectious diseases. I sensed he didn't like me from the start.

"Five years in Africa. That's a long time. Why did you stay so long?"

"I enjoyed it. I got a lot of satisfaction out of what I did there and didn't want to leave until the job was done."

"You probably had a big house there."

"No, it was very small. Only three rooms built of cement blocks."

"Swimming pool?"

"No, but there were some in the American community which everyone could use."

"How often did you?"

"Never actually. I don't know how to swim."

"They certainly must have paid you a lot of money to work in a place like that."

153

"Not all that much, but it was enough for me."

"Well you must have gotten bonuses and allowances."

"Five hundred dollars a year for cost of living."

He scanned my résumé. "You've written a lot of papers in medical journals about infectious diseases in Africa. But I see you've written some on native customs."

"Yes, I have. I'm an amateur anthropologist."

"You must have spent a lot of time studying native dances and customs."

"Not much. Mostly at night when I was in villages. There wasn't anything to do. So I would interview the old men and study traditional medicine and sculpture and dances."

He got up from behind his desk and said he wanted to show me the infectious-disease service in the hospital. We walked down the hall to the medical wards. The interns and residents were at the nursing station, writing up charts.

"This is Dr. Imperato," he said, without bothering to introduce them to me by name. "He's just back from five years in Africa. It's five years, isn't it?" he asked, turning to me.

"Yes, five years."

"Dr. Imperato spent a lot of time studying native dances and customs and getting a tan at the ambassador's swimming pool." He laughed and then slapped me on the back. "Just a little joke, son."

He told the resident that he wanted to show me a patient who had been admitted with meningococcal meningitis. The resident pulled the chart and we all walked down the hall to the patient's room.

"How are you today, dear?" he asked the sixteen-year-old girl. She was propped up in a comfortable bed in a private room whose wide window gave a view of the New York skyline.

"Much better." She smiled back.

"She had meningococcal meningitis," he said. "She was far gone when she came in, but I pulled her through. Didn't I, sweetie?" he said, patting her on the leg. She smiled back, but the resident and interns, who no doubt did all the work treating this girl, didn't look happy with his remark.

The resident presented the case like memorized lines of poetry.

"It's a rare disease," my host said. "You've probably never seen a case, have you?"

154

"As a matter of fact, I have. A number of cases."

"But not as difficult as this one?"

"Worse."

I could see that he was getting angry. I was upstaging him in front of his staff. But he had set himself up and I didn't hold back any punches. I had decided before we left his office that I couldn't work for him.

"How many cases have you seen?" he asked me.

"A couple of thousand."

It was a bombshell and the interns and residents glared at me in disbelief. So I told them about the Bamako epidemic and purposely went into great detail, describing the meningitis belt in West Africa.

Everywhere I went for interviews my African experience was treated not only with curiosity, but more importantly, with suspicion. They weren't interested so much in what I had done, but rather in why I had done it. I even went so far as to purge my résumé of my nonmedical papers, which at the time numbered less than a dozen. I submitted only my medical research papers. But that had little effect.

I had some time before arranged to see a former college professor of mine, Dr. C. William Lacaillade, chairman of the Biology Department at St. John's University. Dr. Lacaillade had trained at Harvard and had conducted his early research at the Rockefeller Institute. He was an eminent parasitologist and had strongly encouraged me to pursue my interest in tropical medicine and work in Africa. Over the years we became very close friends and corresponded regularly all the time I was in Mali. He was close to the medical profession, having served as the chairman of the premedical advisory at St. John's for many years. I told him about my experiences.

He was understanding. "But I'm not surprised," he said. "They can't understand someone like yourself who has done the unusual. Your career has been such a dramatic departure from the norm, something completely alien to most of them. And unfortunately, instead of commending you for it, they are condemning you. But that's because their own views are extremely parochial."

"Why are they so down on my avocations?"

"Because they themselves have few interests outside of medi-

155

cine. They've been conditioned to think that if you don't give all of your time to medicine you're in some way less of a physician.''

"But many of them play golf, don't they?"

"Certainly they do. And you would be more credible to them if you had played golf in Africa instead of conducting ethnographic studies in your spare time. You've got to realize too,'' he went on, "that many of them have the erroneous view that Americans who work overseas are either there for the money or because they are dropouts from society here.''

The long and short of it was that my years in Africa weren't a foundation upon which I could build the next stage of my career. From the perspective of today, I see that those years, while full of rewarding and valuable experiences, were so unique as to place them outside the continuum of what went before and what would follow. Some of the skills and knowledge which I acquired in Africa would prove useful later on, but the totality of experience simply wasn't the visa to a future as I had anticipated. It took me quite a long time to accept this reality because it seemed to me harsh and unfair. It wasn't really, as I came to see much later on. And so I decided to start all over again, with trepidation and mixed feelings, but with the resolve that I would succeed.

In making this fresh start, I was greatly aided by a number of people. My former professor of public health, Dr. Duncan Clark, counseled me to begin a career in epidemiology here in the United States.

"They're looking for a chief epidemiologist and director of the Bureau of Infectious Diseases at the City Health Department,'' he told me. "That would be a superb position for you. You would gain enormous experience, establish working professional relationships with colleagues all over the country and become known in the field.''

I was tantalized, but I wasn't ready to jump at the opportunity. As great as this position sounded, I weighed and measured it through the optic of my prejudices. Angry I may have been with the prejudices of others, but as far as my own prejudices were concerned I was pretty efficient in maintaining them. Among them was an attitude cultivated at home and in schools that working for the city government was for those who couldn't make it anywhere else. City employees had always been portrayed as incompetent, lazy, dumb and uncaring. The comment "He works for the city" wasn't a compliment. It was the Bronx cheer.

I had little direct experience to draw upon. As a sixteen-year-old I had gone to a Health Department center to have a physical examination for my working papers. A group of us were herded into a small room, told to take our shirts off and fill out some forms. I remember we had to write against the wall since there was only a chair in the room. The physician came into the room like Gang Busters. There was scarcely any space for him. He sat down on the chair, collected our papers and then took us one by one. His physical examinations consisted of a few quick touches with the stethoscope which I realize from my subsequent training couldn't have picked up even one full beat of a heart. And then he fired off some quick questions which we had trouble understanding because he spoke with such a thick accent. As we stood in front of the chair he told us to drop our pants and then telling us to cough he gave us a few quick pokes in the genitals. "Okay, get out, you're finished," he shouted, barely giving us time to pull up our trousers.

The physicians in my family didn't hold Health Department doctors in high esteem nor did most people I had ever spoken to. Although there were many competent and conscientious doctors working for the department, there were also some who were mediocre. The department was the refuge of those who couldn't make it on the outside. But what many people didn't know was that the department also possessed superb quality in its medical staff. Those physicians, however, weren't always in the front lines, interfacing with the ordinary citizen. The doctor with the thick accent who spoke to us gruffly and who shoved us out the door with our pants half off was the kind of person who gave the department its lasting public image.

Dr. Clark told me to contact Dr. Lowell Bellin, the First Deputy Commissioner of Health. I waited a few days before doing so. In the interim I spoke with people about the possibility of being the chief epidemiologist for the city. The reaction was consistent and predictable.

"What? Work for the city? You've got to be crazy," one of my friends said.

"But I'll be the chief epidemiologist."

"Doesn't matter. The Mrs. Papuffnicks of the world won't know

157

that. But they will know that you're a Board of Health doctor."

"The Board of Health has nothing to do with it. It's a legislative body which makes laws which are incorporated into the Health Code."

He laughed. "You're too much. Tell that to Mrs. Papuffnick. Board of Health, Health Department, it's all the same. You'll be branded a loser and a political hack. And by the way, how is this guy Clark going to get you this job? Does he have political connections?"

"Political connections?"

"Yeah. You know, clubhouse stuff and all that."

"That's got nothing to do with it," I said, amazed that someone would even think that way.

"Tell that to Mrs. Papuffnick too." He laughed. "She'll never believe it."

"These jobs aren't political," I insisted. He didn't believe me, nor did most people. This erroneous conception became more of an irritant to me when I was appointed Commissioner of Health in late 1976 by Mayor Abraham Beame. Many assumed wrongly that the appointment was "political" and in so doing inferred that it wasn't made on the basis of professional competency. As far as they were concerned it was made either because I had political connections, which I didn't, or because it was a political reward for my supposed political efforts on the mayor's behalf. What they didn't know or care to accept was that I and all of my immediate predecessors were chosen because whoever was mayor was convinced we could handle an extremely complex job requiring skill and experience. Search committees were established composed of leading public-health experts and a selection made only after careful consideration. Before Mayor Beame appointed me in 1976, he consulted with a number of public-health experts and with leaders in medicine such as Martin Begun, the associate dean of the New York University School of Medicine, and Dr. Howard Rusk. What many people didn't know was that Dean Begun and Dr. Rusk were vital creative forces in the public-health affairs of the city who provided the mayor with valuable counsel on a number of difficult problems. During my three years as First Deputy Commissioner I got to know both of these men and sought their advice on many issues. In later years I would tell people that I became Commissioner of Health of New York City because of the strong recommendations made to the mayor by my predecessor, Dr. Lowell Bellin, by Dean Begun, Dr. Howard Rusk and other public-health experts and they would continue to disbelieve me!

I finally called Dr. Bellin, a man whom I didn't know at the time, but one who would shape my career as no one else ever has.

"Lowell Bellin here," he said over the phone.

"Dr. Clark suggested I call you about the position of chief epidemiologist."

"Oh, yes," Bellin replied with enthusiasm. "When can you come in?"

"How about tomorrow?"

"Fine, come in at one P.M. My office is in room 332."

Bellin was a tall man with an enormous amount of energy, like a piece of burning lava shot out of a volcano. We took an instant liking to one another. He read through my résumé, that is, the purged version, and then he said, smiling, "This is fantastic. You've got a master's from Tulane, a residency in internal medicine, CDC training. Excellent."

He pressed the intercom. "Please ask Dr. Chaves to come over."

I had a good feeling about this interview because it was unlike many of the others I had been through. Clearly, Bellin didn't feel threatened by me as some of the others had. His candid assessments, his unassuming manner and splendid reputation told me that this was an exceptional man.

Dr. Aaron Chaves was the Assistant Commissioner for Chronic and Communicable Diseases. Although I had never met him, I knew of him because he was one of the leading authorities on tuberculosis in the United States. Bellin handed him my résumé. He read it over page by page, occasionally looking up at me. Bellin sat at the head of the conference table, beaming like a cat that had just swallowed the canary. Only later would I learn why. At that time he and others were dismayed by the deprofessionalization which had occurred in the Health Services Administration, the Mayor Lindsay–created super-agency in which the Health Department was located. Young college students without experience or training were often given major responsibilities which they couldn't handle. Their failures were easily submerged within the thick layers of

159

a big bureaucracy but they were a daily nightmare for professionals like Bellin and Chaves who had to live with them. It was a joy for Bellin to be able to recruit a professional, and the fact that he himself had worked overseas in the Negev Desert, rendering health care to the Bedouins, equipped him to understand someone like myself.

"Duncan Clark thinks he's great," Bellin said to Chaves right in front of me. Both Chaves and I smiled. I didn't know then that Bellin was also a Downstate graduate and that Dr. Clark had been his professor as well.

Chaves kept reading the résumé. Then he looked up and said, "You have an impressive background and we are interested in you."

Bellin said he had to go to a meeting and jumped up from his chair. "You handle him, Aaron. Check him out and all that." And then turning toward me he said, "I hope you will be able to join us. It will be the experience of a lifetime." Little did I know how right he was.

Chaves arranged for me to meet with the Commissioner of Health, Dr. Mary McLaughlin, and with one of the Deputy Commissioners, Dr. Warren Toff. Whatever reservaticns I had about working for the department were erased after meeting these four public-health physicians. I looked forward to hearing from Dr. Chaves and hoped the response would be favorable.

Dr. Chaves called three days later. "The job is yours."

I almost couldn't believe it. "Thanks. Thanks."

"When do you want to start?"

"Start? Yes, start. January? Is January all right?"

"Fine with us," Chaves replied. "I'll process your papers."

CHAPTER 13

BREAKING INTO NEW YORK CITY

The Health Department building is an imposing gray granite cube ten stories high, essentially Grecian but with a strong dash of Art Deco. It stands on the north side of Foley Square in the downtown section of Manhattan, not far from City Hall. Foley Square is famous because of the courts which flank one side of it. Indictments, trials, convictions and acquittals take place in them every day and are a magnet to newsmen, TV crews and radio reporters. Across from them is the giant modern Federal Building, a skyscraper which towers above all its neighbors, and at the southern tip of the square stands the Municipal Building, another giant Grecian temple with archways and an inner court. By chance, the Health Department building occupies a choice spot in this modern forum. Its southern exposure gives it sun most of the day and a superb view of the triangular park with its sycamore trees and exhibits of giant modern sculptures.

The frieze around the top of the building is etched with the names of famous men of medicine and public health—Jenner, Koch, Pineal, Biggs, Hippocrates, Ramazzini and many others. They span centuries. I looked up at them. It was an impressive sight.

I reported to Dr. Chaves's office on the third floor.

"Let's go up," he said. "I'll introduce you to the staff of the bureau."

The bureau was housed in a suite of rooms, partitioned from ceiling to floor by metal and frosted glass. They hadn't made partitions that way in a long time. Both they and the walls needed a painting badly. They were covered with a dull green which was smothered with several layers of dust and grime. The floor still had the original brown linoleum dating to 1933 when the building was completed. It and the old wall fans, battered desks and bleached window shades had long since proven their durability. What a dismal place! As Chaves took me around I kept thinking to myself, what did I ever get into? The bureau reeked of the past. It seemed to me it had stood still for at least a quarter of a century while time marched on.

Chaves introduced me to the staff. Some of them were old-timers who had been there for years doing the same routine day after day. It was familiar and secure and they didn't want it changed. It's the instinctual reaction of most long-entrenched bureaucrats to react to a young newcomer with suspicion, especially if he is in a position to initiate change. My smiles and handshakes and inane chitchat didn't seem to cut the ice with them. They glared at me with somber faces from behind desks piled high with papers and files. I wondered to myself how necessary all those papers were to the control of communicable diseases in the city. It didn't occur to me that I had little experience in working in a complex bureaucracy. Nor did I understand, as I would in later years, why the old-timers were suspicious of change. Time and again, they had seen yesterday's administrative heresies presented as modern innovations.

"This is Tom Murray," Chaves said, introducing me to a short, rotund man in shirtsleeves. "He's your office manager and will be your right-hand man."

"Nice to meet you," I said, shaking hands. He smiled a bit nervously, sizing me up, and then sensing no danger, broke into a broad grin and poured out, "We're here to help you, Doctor. Need anything? Just ask. We'll do our best to deliver." The accent wasn't pure Brooklynese. Somewhere at a crucial age he had moved to the Bronx.

"Are you from the Bronx?" I asked.

"Yeah, howd'you know?"

"Easy. I recognize the accent."

He laughed. "Boy, you're sharp. But you know, I wasn't born there. I grew up in Brooklyn."

We chatted about Brooklyn and the Bronx. It wasn't the same in either place, he said. He had moved out to the island like everybody else.

"We're sure glad they found somebody for this here job, Doctor. Ain't many of you epidemiologist guys around anymore."

Chaves looked a bit pained. "Let's go on," he said, steering me toward a far end of the suite. Murray followed tenaciously behind.

"We've only got five clerks, Doctor," he bellowed. Chaves and I turned around. He raised his arms to add emphasis and jerked them up and down. "But we need ten."

"Why do you need so many?" I asked.

His right arm swept out toward the huge dingy room where I had just seen the heaps of papers and files every color of the rainbow.

"We gotta process all the forms, you know." There was a glint in his eye.

"Uh, let's not get into that just yet, Tom," Chaves replied. "Some other time."

"But I gotta have them there clerks, Doctor," Murray came back with emphasis and determination.

"We'll talk about it later," Chaves said.

"Let me show you your office." He paced off toward a doorway and I followed him.

"This is it," he said, smiling and looking anxious about my reaction. It was in a corner with two windows, one on the park and the other facing a deserted loft building with broken windows. Compared to my Bamako office, it was Park Avenue and I had no reason to complain. Chaves apologized for the dust.

"The Public Works people are responsible for cleaning. But they don't do a very good job of it."

The dust didn't bother me. What did was the unused look to the place.

"When did the last director leave?"

"Four months ago," bellowed Murray from the doorway before Chaves could reply. "That's right, it was about four months ago," said Chaves.

163

"I'm tellin' you, Dr. Chaves, we're sure lucky Dr. Imperato took this here job because me and the girls out there couldn't handle it much longer."

There was no stopping Murray. "We can't get doctors to work for this here department like before. The city don't pay much. Not compared to what you can make in practice."

Chaves interrupted. "What Tom means is that our salaries aren't competitive with the private sector. It's extremely difficult to get physicians to work for a public-health department in a place like New York because of the quality of life, cost of living and high state and city income taxes."

"You can sure say that again," Murray piped in. "Wait till you see what they take out in them taxes. I'll bet you didn't pay state and city taxes in Africa."

"No I didn't," I said. "I didn't have to since I was living overseas."

"Well, now they'll hit you for twenty percent on top of the Federal."

"I want to introduce Dr. Imperato to Dr. Herbert," said Chaves, interrupting.

Bill Herbert was the Epidemic Intelligence Service officer assigned by the CDC to New York City. He was the only full-time epidemiologist in the department. That came as a surprise to me. During the four months that the bureau had been without a director he had been running things pretty much alone. The only other full-time physician was Dr. Theodore Hinkle, a sixty-nine-year-old career Health Department physician who Herbert told me had been retired to the bureau to keep him out of trouble.

"Senile?"

"I think so," Herbert said.

"He's a garbage-picker," boomed Murray. "Why, every lunch hour he goes out with two shopping bags and picks through the garbage cans up near Canal Street. Come on, I'll show you," he said, motioning us to a narrow office nearby.

"Look at this," Murray said, opening the door on Hinkle's private hideaway. It was stacked with old magazines, newspapers, broken furniture, clothes hangers, textile cuttings stuffed into over a score of plastic bags and an assortment of old equipment including television sets which didn't work and three air conditioners missing most of their inners.

164

"I don't know how he gets the stuff up here," Murray said.

Chaves had already left and I found shutting Murray up a difficult job. He could ramble on for hours. It wasn't even ten A.M. and already I felt as if I had been in the bureau twenty years. The ghost of epidemiology past gripped the place.

Ida Peters, my secretary, was out that day, so I didn't meet her until the following morning. She had been in the Health Department thirty-five years and had worked for Morris Greenberg, who was the leading epidemiologist in the country back in the 1950s when he headed the bureau. Ida was as good an epidemiologist as anyone I had ever met. She had been around some of the best all her working life. She knew how to triage reports, to ferret out the important from the routine and to follow up on leads which often led to the cracking of a difficult case.

The bureau had four divisions and Epidemiology was but one of them. The other three were the division of Tropical Medicine, the Veterinary Division and the Immunization Program. Besides Bill Herbert and Ida, there was no other full-time staff in Epidemiology. But there were twenty-five part-time physicians who worked a session or so per day investigating cases. According to Murray a session was two and a half hours.

"They rake in around fifteen grand a year. That's half of what you get. And they only work two and a half hours a day."

When Murray told me this I asked him why it was so.

"The City can't hire full-time people. Full-time salaries like yours are too low. But them part-time salaries are something else. They ain't under civil service regulations. So the department can pay a part-time person more."

I got it, all right. But it seemed to me eminently unfair for them to be earning half my salary for working a quarter of the time I did.

"That's the way it is," Murray said. "That's why I told Chaves he was sure lucky to get you to take this here job."

The Epidemiology Division had vacant lines—that is, open positions for full-time epidemiologists. But the salaries offered under civil service were so low that the bureau hadn't been able to fill them in years.

"No point in having those lines," Herbert said to me. "Nobody's going to come and work as an epidemiologist for twenty thousand a year."

And for that the city's Department of Personnel required that applicants have an M.D. degree, a master's degree in public health, a New York State license to practice medicine and five years' experience in epidemiology! It wasn't just the linoleum and the fans which were out of date. The civil service requirements for these positions had been put on the books back in the 1950s and so had the salaries. The bureau was in desperate need of epidemiologists. Something had to be done. Either the salaries had to be increased to attract physician epidemiologists or else I had to come up with a plan to train and hire nonphysician epidemiologists. I wasn't sure what I was going to do. Even that first horrifying day I thought about training public-health nurses as epidemiologists. But getting something new and innovative like that through the city's bureaucracy would take years. It did, but eventually fifteen nurse epidemiologists came on board to replace the part-time doctors and fill in for the physician epidemiologists I was never able to hire.

"You're lucky Dr. Shookhoff is in charge of the Tropical Division," Herbert went on. "You won't have to worry about it."

The Division of Tropical Medicine ran four clinics, treating about ten thousand people a year, mostly poor immigrants from Latin America and the Caribbean who were suffering from parasitic diseases. Dr. Howard Shookhoff, the chief of this division, was one of the leading authorities in the United States on tropical medicine, and he directed a superb staff of part-time and full-time specialists.

Likewise the Immunization Program, funded by the CDC, was administered by public-health advisors who were excellent. It and the Tropical-disease Division were alive and well. But Epidemiology and the Veterinary Division were in sad shape. Department regulars called the Veterinary Division the dog-bite bureau because it handled the forty thousand reported dog bites in the city.

I met the chief of the division the first day. He had been with the department for over thirty years.

"They're trying to destroy the Veterinary Division," he said when we first met.

"Who's the they?" I asked.

"The higher-ups."

"Why would they want to do that?"

"I don't really know. All I know is that they're trying to destroy us."

166

Dr. Malcolm Todd ran his division from regulations which had been put on the books in the 1920s. Epidemiology may have existed in the fifties, but veterinary public health was operating in an even earlier period. Todd had a full-time sidekick by the name of Arthur Latimer, Ph.D., D.Sc. He and Todd spent most of their time in court and when they weren't there they held hearings and passed out fines with the help of four policemen assigned to the division by the Police Department. The cops were on what was called limited duty since they had some kind of physical disability.

In addition to Latimer, Todd had several part-time veterinarians working for him. Their job was to examine the ten thousand dogs brought into the ASPCA shelters each year and to make sure they didn't have rabies. Every time a dog bit someone, the treating physician or hospital emergency room sent in a report on a yellow card known in the bureau as the "395." Upon receipt of this card, Todd's clerks sent a letter to the dog owner, if known, telling him to take his dog to the ASPCA shelter in his borough to be examined for the possible presence of rabies. Among the forty thousand people whose bites were reported to Todd's division in any given year, dogs and their owners were identified in only ten thousand. That meant that thirty thousand dogs were never examined, not to mention the ones that bit people who didn't even report their bites.

Dog owners who complied with the order for the examination were given a card to return for a follow-up examination in four weeks. And if they complied with both examinations, the veterinarian sent a white form to the central office closing the case out. If they didn't comply, the veterinarian sent a large blue form to the central office and they in turn sent out a blue reminder card to the dog owner. If the dog owner didn't show up at the shelter with the dog within four weeks, a follow-up notice was sent out on a pink card. Failure to respond to any of these reminders elicited a visit from Todd's policemen. But since there were only four of them they couldn't get to all of the noncomplying dog owners.

"There hasn't been any rabies in either dogs or cats in this city in over twenty-five years," I told Todd many weeks later. "Why do you bother examining all these dogs?"

"That's how we prevent it, Dr. Imperato." Todd spoke slowly, deliberately and always courteously. But I didn't see his logic.

"At most you examine only ten thousand out of the forty thousand dogs which bite people in any given year. You don't see the other thirty thousand."

"Doesn't matter. That's how we prevent rabies."

"But how?"

"I don't really know, Dr. Imperato. I can only tell you that we're successful at it."

I had by then studied up on rabies in New York City and saw logic to the present system when it was first instituted at the turn of the century when rabies was rampant in the dog and cat populations in the city. Veterinarians were able to diagnose rabies in biting animals and victims were then treated quickly and their lives saved. But the disease had been absent from the city's dog and cat population for over a quarter of a century, mainly because of high levels of immunity in these animal populations from vaccination. Also, there is virtually no rabies in the wildlife populations living in rural areas adjacent to the city. Where rabies is present in the United States in dog and cat populations, it usually gets there by spread from infected wild animals such as skunks, foxes and raccoons.

Todd's elaborate bureaucratic procedures and examinations were in a sense a waste of time. None of this prevented rabies. It only confirmed the continued absence of the disease. The procedures had to be changed, but there was no convincing Todd.

"They're trying to destroy the Veterinary Division, Dr. Imperato," he would reply. "I know. I've been around a long time."

No one was trying to destroy the division. But I did want to change it and update its procedures. I was finally able to accomplish this, but it took a couple of years and a lot of hard fighting within the bureaucracy. Today the Health Department examines fewer than a thousand dogs a year and fewer than a dozen people receive antirabies treatment compared to the two thousand who did before. Those who do today are people bitten overseas or in areas of the United States where rabies is present.

On my second day on the job, Ida Peters came in to tell me that an irate woman was on the phone demanding to speak to the director.

"Her daughter has head lice, Doctor. And Dr. Hinkle told her to dust her head with DDT powder."

"DDT?"

168

Ida opened her eyes wide. "I know, isn't that terrible?"

"Hasn't Hinkle ever read *Silent Spring*?"

"I guess not. Anyway this woman went to a hardware store and asked for DDT powder. The salesman told her it was banned by the Food and Drug Administration."

"What happened then?"

"The salesman told her that Health Department doctors are incompetent."

In this case the salesman was right. Hinkle was a menace, an old man who refused to retire and who was in a pension plan which permitted him to work until seventy. Even that pension plan had been retired twenty years before. But to get him out via civil service procedures would have required almost a year. And I wasn't sure I would succeed because he had lucid periods when he was coherent, intelligent and in full command of his judgment capabilities. And then there were times when he was completely out of it.

"I'll speak with the woman, Ida, but find Dr. Hinkle for me."

When Ida returned five minutes later she came with Murray in tow.

"He's probably up on Canal Street getting more cuttings," he hollered. "Did you see that No Parking sign he hauled in yesterday?"

I hadn't seen Hinkle's latest acquisition and I wasn't interested in seeing it either. But I told Murray and Ida that no calls from the public or from physicians were to be given to Dr. Hinkle. He was to be restricted to sorting reports and records of cases scheduled for filing.

As they left, Bill Herbert came in with several sheets of yellow legal paper.

"I think we have a salmonella outbreak," he said. "Six cases have been reported by private physicians over the past two days."

"How do you know it's an outbreak?"

"I didn't at first. But then on speaking with each of the six I learned that they had all been to a wedding reception in Queens. Er, yeah, let's see," he went on, flipping through the sheets. "Crotona Palace. That's the name of the place."

"Incubation period right?" I asked.

"Yeah, eight to twenty-four hours and they all had severe diarrhea and fever."

169

"Have they eaten together anywhere else in the past several days?"

"No. In fact two of the people are from the the groom's side and don't know the other four from the bride's family."

There was pretty strong evidence pointing to what epidemiologists call "a common source" of infection, meaning that all of these people were exposed to the same contaminated food at about the same time. Salmonella causes gastroenteritis. There are over seventy types of this bacterium.

"Are you getting stool specimens from the six?"

"Yeah, the drivers went out already for them. The lab should have results for us by the end of the week."

"If it's the same type in all six then it's almost certain they got it at the wedding reception."

But almost certain wasn't the same as certain in epidemiologic jargon. We had to find the food which was contaminated and then snoop some more and find out how it got contaminated. Was it by a food handler at the Crotona Palace? Or did the food come already contaminated from the wholesaler? If it had been contaminated in production, then many lots coming out of the factory might be infected and outbreaks would occur all over the place. Finding the source of the infection had more than just local implications.

"I've gotten the name of the bride's family. They gave the reception and if they can give me a list of the guests I can call them and find out how many got sick."

Bill Herbert sighed a bit. "And then—and then I'll have to find out which foods the sick people ate that the well people didn't."

"It's a tedious way to pinpoint it," I said. "But maybe we can speed it up if we have the sanitary inspectors go out to the place and take samples of foods there. That might turn something up."

Herbert looked skeptical.

"I know it's a long shot. Maybe the food's been discarded. But it's worth a try."

Herbert smiled as he walked out. "Okay. You're the boss."

Miss Parthenia Pebbles was the sanitary inspector assigned to the bureau for food-outbreak investigations. She was about fifty, a short, trim woman who dressed in neatly pressed suits, blouses with bows and ruffles and a hat.

170

"Hard as nails," Murray had described her to me. "Don't let that finishing-school getup fool you."

I didn't find her hard as nails, but she was thorough, tenacious and meticulously organized in conducting an investigation.

I gave her the facts and she copied everything down on a small pad in tiny letters resembling the footnotes in a medieval manuscript.

"Anything else?" she asked quietly.

"No, I think that's it. Dr. Herbert is trying to locate the bride's family and get a list of the guests."

She nodded approvingly. "This is a good start. I will go out to the Crotona Palace with two of my assistants and will call you from there." She looked at her watch. "I should have some information for you at about three P.M."

After Miss Pebbles left, Bill Herbert came back looking exasperated. "Wow. That bride's mother is really ticked off. She won't cooperate nohow."

"She won't give you the list of guests?"

"That's right. Says she doesn't have it. Her daughter supposedly has it and she's away on her honeymoon and no one knows where she is."

"Likely story."

"Yeah, sounds phony to me," Herbert replied.

"Maybe I ought to give it a try," I said.

"Fine," Bill replied. "Here's her number."

Norbertina Bacigalupo. The name itself was formidable. I dialed the number as Herbert stood by on the extension.

"Hello." She didn't have the accent I expected.

"Mrs. Bacigalupo?"

"Yes."

"My name is Dr. Imperato. I'm with the New York City Health Department."

She cut me off. "I just spoke with a doctor from the Board of Health. There was nothing wrong with my daughter's wedding reception. My husband and I gave her the best wedding reception money can buy. I ate everything at the reception and so did my husband and we didn't get sick."

"Mrs. Bacigalupo, I understand that your daughter's reception was a very lovely affair. But six people have become ill and we

171

think they may have eaten something at the reception. We can't say for sure. That's why we need your help."

I got nowhere with her. "I can't help you. I don't know anything. My daughter planned her own wedding reception and she has the list. She's in the Poconos now."

At that Bill Herbert looked up and smiled.

"Poconos?" I asked.

"No, maybe it's the Catskills. I don't know."

"Mrs. Bacigalupo, we need your help. Won't you please give us the list of guests? All we want to do is call them and ask them if they've been sick with diarrhea recently."

"I'm not giving you any list. I don't have it and that's that. I'm not going to have you calling four hundred people and telling them that I served poisoned food at my daughter's reception."

"No one is saying you served bad food," I replied.

"That's what they'll say. And I'm suspicious that those Esposito people did this to me."

"Esposito people?"

"Yeah. Did any of those six people go by the name of Esposito?"

Bill nodded no.

"I don't think so," I said to her.

"Well I think so. I didn't want to invite them. They're distant relatives of my husband and we don't get along. It got back to me at the reception what they were saying."

"What were they saying?"

"That my Philomena's reception wasn't as nice as their Millie's. They're trying to smear me up, that's what it is. Well I'm not going to stand for it. I didn't want them, but he insisted. Now look at all the trouble they've made for me."

"Mrs. Bacigalupo, I don't think they are trying to make any trouble for you. No one by that name is on our list of sick people."

"They probably got someone else to say they're sick. That's what they did. Well I'll fix them. Just you wait. I'll teach them a lesson they'll never forget."

"Mrs. Bacigalupo, please, I think—" I heard a click.

"She hung up," Bill said from across the room, holding up the dead receiver.

"Too bad. We're only trying to help," he added.

172

"I guess you can't blame her for not wanting us to tell all her friends and relatives that there was a problem at the reception. It was probably the most important social occasion of her life and she could never live with what she would see as an enormous disgrace." I was sensitive to Mrs. Bacigalupo's feelings, but we had to get at the source of the outbreak. I called the manager of the Crotona Palace.

"We're not allowed to give out such confidential information," the manager told me. "We are honor bound to protect the privacy of our clients at all times."

"Another dead end," I muttered. My only recourse now was to subpoena the list from Mrs. Bacigalupo. But I didn't want to do that unless there was stronger evidence. And there was still the possibility that we would turn up the source without contacting the guests at the reception. True, the investigation would be less complete. But the important thing now was to track down the source and eliminate it.

At three P.M. sharp Miss Pebbles called. "I have inspected the entire kitchen and food-preparation areas," she said. "Inadequate drainage in one sink, poor lighting in one freezer, dust on the lighting fixtures and grease stains on wall tiles beneath the stove."

"She must have gotten down on all fours to have found that last one," I said to myself.

"Anything else?"

"Yes. There are a number of food remainders still in the freezer and I have taken samples of all of them. There are twenty-six in all. I have confiscated and condemned all of them. Is there anything else you want me to do here?"

"No, I can't think of anything."

"Very well. In that case, I will proceed directly to the laboratories and have the food specimens tested. We should have some answers by Friday."

At the laboratory, the food samples were streaked out on plates containing a waxy-looking material on which bacteria, especially salmonella, grow very well. On Friday morning, Miss Pebbles called me.

"We have found salmonella, Dr. Imperato. In the liver pâté. All the other foods are negative. We should know the type by Monday."

173

At last we had a break. So it was the liver pâté. Miss Pebbles and Bill Herbert went back out to the Crotona Palace to find out how it was prepared and who handled it. Somehow the pâté had gotten infected with salmonella.

Miss Pebbles called at noon to say that the pâté was mixed on the premises by a cook, William Smith.

"I suspect he contaminated it," she said, "But of course I cannot be sure."

"We had better get stool cultures on all the cooks, kitchen hands and waiters. How many are there?"

"Thirty-three," she replied. "Dr. Imperato, I already ordered all of them to the labs for cultures when I was here on Friday and all of them showed up there this morning."

"Oh, very good," I said. Boy, was she efficient.

"Smith is back here now and I plan to interrogate him."

What an interrogation! Bill Herbert later told me that she cross-examined him without mercy. Then he broke. Yes, he had stuck his fingers into the pâté as he mixed it. But only to taste it to make sure the consistency and flavor were right.

She didn't flinch when she asked him about his personal toilet habits. Sure, he washed his hands after he wiped himself.

"Absolutely sure?" she asked.

"Yeah."

"You didn't forget even once? Most of us do. I'm sure you are no different from the rest of us."

"Oh, maybe I forgot a couple of times. You know, it's busy and the boss wants you to get the food out fast. You know how it is."

"Of course I do," Miss Pebbles replied.

Two days later, on Wednesday, Miss Pebbles called from the laboratories. "*Salmonella newport* in the six cases, in the pâté and in Mr. Smith's stool. All the other workers are negative.

"You've solved it, Miss Pebbles. Congratulations!"

"It is very kind of you, Dr. Imperato. But it is just part of my job."

Smith was carrying *Salmonella newport* in his intestinal tract and injected it into the liver pâté with his finger after he came out of the john. The pâté was a good substance for the microbe to grow in, especially when it was brought out to be served on the buffet table.

174

The warmer room temperatures created a more favorable climate for it to multiply at a rapid rate. Salmonella organisms don't multiply very rapidly under refrigeration, but they do survive.

Bill Herbert was unhappy about not being able to interview all the people who attended the reception.

"I could have gotten food histories from them, made up a list of foods the sick people ate versus the ones the well people ate and arrived at a conclusion about which food was responsible."

"Maybe," I said, "but probably not. People at a wedding reception eat so much, they usually can't remember what they've had off a buffet table. And besides, some who ate the pâté when it was first put out might not have gotten sick."

"How could that be?" he asked.

"Because there may not have been a high enough concentration of microorganisms present at that time to cause diarrhea. With each passing hour the bacteria multiplied at a geometric rate, reaching concentrations which made people sick when they ate the pâté."

"So that's why you wanted Pebbles to get hold of the foods."

"Sure, it's the fastest way to pinpoint the source in a food-borne outbreak. Doing it through a process of elimination like you wanted is valid and the only recourse when the foods have been thrown out. But often you end up with not being able to tag the contaminated food."

Bill shook his head. "Isn't that something. You learn something new every day in this business.

"But tell me," he added, "where did Smith get infected?"

"Hard to say. *Newport* is a common type. He could have gotten it anywhere."

He leaned over on the desk. "And another thing. Why wasn't he sick?"

"Probably was, but it may have been so mild he didn't take notice. Or maybe he had a bad diarrhea and doesn't want to own up to it."

"Do you think he got it in Newport, Rhode Island?" Bill laughed.

I laughed too. "Maybe, but I doubt it."

We kept Smith under surveillance for several weeks. He was not permitted to go back to work until three consecutive stool examinations were negative, confirming he was free from infection.

"I have instructed him in hand washing," Miss Pebbles said over the phone several days later. "And I have told him that I will be checking up on him at the Crotona Palace." And she did.

CHAPTER 14

NEOPHYTE ADMINISTRATOR

News travels fast within the Health Department and in a few weeks a delegation came to see me from the Municipal Union of Physicians, Surgeons and Dentists. They came in blasting threats and invectives, all based on the flimsy rumor that I was out to destroy the bureau. The ill-defined "they" Todd and the others always spoke about had now narrowed down to me.

The meeting started off with a presentation of their strength.

"Over a thousand members," the leader of the group said, "and we've struck before."

"What are you trying to tell me?" I replied.

The leader didn't want to be candid. He had been speaking in obfuscations for so many years he just couldn't come to the point.

"We want to do everything possible to help you bring better services to the people of the city," he said.

I didn't really believe him.

"And to do that you need the support of our physicians."

I nodded approvingly.

"We understand that you are reorganizing the bureau and intend to eliminate vital services, lifesaving services"—he raised his voice—"for the people of the city. We can't stand by and allow the health of the city to be jeopardized."

"I don't plan to eliminate anything that is vital to the health of the city. I do plan, however, to introduce some efficiency into the operations of the bureau."

"Efficiency!" another member of the delegation shouted. "That's what they always call it. It's just another name for wiping out jobs."

He shocked me with his candor. I hadn't expected the real agenda to surface until at least another hour of beating around the bush.

"Nurses can't do the work of doctors," the leader said, narrowing the agenda down to the real bone of contention.

"I don't agree with you," I replied. "It's been amply proven that they can do a lot of things people thought were sacred to doctors."

"They can't do epidemiology. Show me where they've done it as good as doctors."

"It's not my job to show you. Go look for yourself in hospitals all over the country and you'll find out."

The meeting went on for another hour. They made it clear they weren't going to stand by and let me bring in nurse epidemiologists to replace the members of their union. I had done my homework before the meeting and found out that less than half of my part-time physician epidemiologists were members of the union.

"Most of the physician epidemiologists are up in years and due to retire soon," I said, "and as you know very well, the bureau hasn't been able to recruit replacements the past few years."

"We're here to protect the rights of our members," the leader replied.

"I thought you said you were interested in the well-being of the people of the city. If you are, then you should be worried about how I'm going to deliver epidemiological services after your members retire to Florida."

"Our members are dedicated men and won't leave the city in the lurch."

"That remains to be seen."

"You have an antidoctor bias," the leader said.

"Oh, come off it," I replied. "How did you ever come up with that one? I have nothing against the physician epidemiologists in this bureau. Most of them are bright and hard-working men. But they're getting old and I've got to plan for the future."

The union was afraid I might fire their members before they be-

178

came eligible to retire on their city pensions. As part-time employees they had all the benefits of civil service except permanency. They were vulnerable to being dismissed at a moment's notice. Once they paid into the pension plan for fifteen years, they could retire. Many of them had two years or so to go to be eligible for their pensions. And I had no doubts that they would follow the pattern of their retired colleagues and quit as soon as they could.

"We want to be part of the planning process," the leader said.

"Fine," I replied. I'll be delighted to have you work with me in putting together a new epidemiology program for the city."

They breathed sighs of relief. Not that they were interested in participating in the planning process. Their aim was to stall me as long as they could. But my offer enabled them to go back to their membership with the claim that there would be no changes in epidemiology to which the union would not agree. For the membership, that meant their jobs were secure.

The constant flow of retirements of aging part-time physicians was draining the union of strength and resolve. I went ahead with my plans, knowing that time was on my side. But right now they had the political clout to checkmate my plans not only at the level of the Health Department but also in the Bureau of the Budget and most importantly at City Hall. I couldn't implement them, not just yet.

Todd and his group had no union representation. Otherwise they would have been in my office every day. Like the part-time epidemiologists, Todd's staff were hard-working and dedicated. But many of the things they did were no longer relevant, and they weren't doing the things which were.

Todd came into my office after the union representatives left. "I have to go up to the Bronx, Dr. Imperato," he said as he shuffled toward my desk. "I have to testify at a court case."

"What's the problem?"

"As you know by now," he said, "the Veterinary Division is crucial to this department."

I nodded yes and cut him off because I had been through this before.

"What's the case about?"

"You see, this man went into the emergency room of Hamford Hospital saying he had been bitten on the nose by one of his pet

179

boa constrictors. They didn't believe him. So he went home and came back with two boas in a box. He opened the box and took them out and let them loose on the floor of the emergency room.''

''What?''

Todd nodded his head. ''Yep, that's what he did.''

''Then what happened?''

''People screamed and jumped up on the tops of tables, chairs and stretchers. They didn't know if the snakes were poisonous or not. Then they called the police.''

Todd looked at the report in his hands. ''Er, it says they arrested him for reckless endangerment.''

''What's going to happen now?''

''Well he has to go before the judge and I've been called as an expert witness.''

''To testify about what?''

''About the snakes. It's against the Health Code regulations to keep snakes in the city like that.'' He stopped for a second and then said, ''Oh, and we're going to fine the pet shop which sold him the snakes.''

I figured that one was coming.

''We're supposed to inspect the pet shops every year. They're over fifteen hundred of them in the city. But Dr. Latimer and I and the staff are so busy with court cases and hearings we don't have the time to go out and do all the inspections.''

''That's the problem,'' I said. ''You shouldn't be involved in all of those court cases and hearings and examining those dogs which don't have rabies. You should be out there inspecting the pet shops and controlling this incredible problem of exotic animals in the city.''

''But the Health Code requires it.''

''The Health Code can be changed.''

''Oh, I wouldn't want to do that, Dr. Imperato.''

''Why not? It's not sacred. The Board of Health is changing sections of it all the time.''

''You can't change the part about animals. It's been there for over fifty years and people won't stand for your tampering with it.''

''If I change it, you and your men will have more time to inspect pet shops. They're selling illegal exotic animals, everything from leopard kittens to snakes."

"And a lot of sick animals too," Todd added. "Look what happened to that poor blind man. You know the one I told you about last week, Dr. Imperato."

"Oh, yes," I remembered. "The one who bought a German shepherd."

Todd nodded and rocked in his chair. "Yes," he said sadly. "And the dog had such bad arthritis it couldn't walk. The poor blind man didn't know it because he can't see."

"That's the kind of thing you should be preventing. Not going to court every day. There are enormous problems with animals in this city, with people buying bigger and more vicious dogs for protection. Some of the lines are badly bred and the animals are extremely vicious. And then look at the problem with guard dogs and attack dogs. Have we done anything about that? No."

Todd replied, "Give me more staff and I'll do something."

"You don't need more staff. All you need is to redeploy your staff. They're wasting all their time examining those healthy dogs which don't have rabies."

"That's how we prevent it, Dr. Imperato."

"Yes, yes, I know, that's how we prevent it." I was exasperated with him. "We don't prevent it. We just confirm it isn't around anymore."

"I don't agree, Dr. Imperato," Todd said timidly. "I'm not trying to be disrespectful, you understand. But the division has prevented rabies in this city for over twenty-five years thanks to the hard work of the veterinarians and people like Dr. Latimer."

"Speaking of Latimer," I interjected, "what has he been doing lately?"

"He's been representing us at the City Council hearings on the proposed bill to make dog owners pick up the poop from the streets."

"For most people, it's an aesthetic problem," I said. "They aren't aware of the *Toxocara* worm infection, which rarely causes serious infections in humans, mainly in the liver and the eye."

"I agree," Todd replied. "Even though the dog haters make it sound like the poop causes all sorts of rampaging epidemics, that

181

doesn't stop dog owners from letting their animals run loose all over the parks. Why just the other day I saw two big Great Danes dropping their poop on the lawn in front of the Hayden Planetarium."

"Obviously the Health Code regulations and the Curb Your Dog signs all over town don't mean anything to these people," I said. "And our sanitary inspectors and the police are so overwhelmed with other problems they don't have the time to follow a dog and catch it in the act of defecating on a sidewalk or in a park."

"Even if they did, it wouldn't do much good," Todd said, "because they would have to catch the owner, who is often down the block or behind some shrubs. You can't hand a summons to a dog, you know," he added laughingly.

The problem of dog litter on the streets and in parks had become a critical one at that time because of the rapid rise in the numbers of dogs in the city. Todd and the staff of the American Society for the Prevention of Cruelty to Animals estimated that there were 700,000 dogs in the city. People were increasingly keeping dogs for protection against crime rather than as pets. This meant that the dogs were larger, more prone to bite and generating more litter than had been the case in the past.

Todd shook his head. "One dog for every ten people. That translates into a lot of dog poop every day!"

Over the weeks, I had come to understand Todd and Latimer and appreciate their good points. They were both conscientious, hard working and sincere and extremely knowledgeable about animals and the problems they caused in a large city like New York. But sometimes they were opinionated, making it difficult for me to get them to change their views on certain issues. The department's handling of dog bites was one of those issues.

We did agree, however, that something had to be done about the dog feces problem. But what? Suggestions poured in every week from private citizens and organized groups, and they ranged from a complete ban on dogs to charging hundreds of dollars a year for a license. Those who proposed the latter said it would discourage people from keeping dogs and didn't agree with us that it would also discriminate against the poor. There were few hard facts about the health hazards of dog feces. A survey conducted some years before in New York City pet shops revealed that 14.5 percent of all the dogs being sold were infected with *Toxocara* worms. But most dogs sold in pet shops are puppies, an important point as far as the *Toxocara* infection is concerned. The worms live in the intestines of dogs; there is also a variety that infects cats. An infected female can pass the infection on to her puppies before they are born. As the puppies grow and mature, the infection dies out and eventually disappears in most.

Those were the only facts we were sure of, and they didn't make a strong case for adult dog poop being a serious health hazard as far as *Toxocara* was concerned. But what did concern Todd and Latimer was the presence of the infection in puppies and the close contact between puppies and children. The adult female *Toxocara* worms, living in the intestines of puppies, lay eggs, which are passed out with the dog's stool. It takes these eggs two weeks to mature. If they are accidentally swallowed before that by someone, nothing happens. But at maturity, these eggs contain a young form of the worm, which hatches out once it reaches a victim's intestinal tract. Children are always putting their fingers and hands into their mouths, and it's easy for them to become infected with these eggs if they're around in a park or even in their own yard at home. Once the worm is in the intestinal tract, it pierces the wall of the bowel and migrates via the blood and lymphatic systems to the liver and lungs. These young worms are known as larvae. Once in the liver, they usually remain there and don't cause much damage in most cases. Those that reach the lungs, however, can then migrate to other parts of the body including the eyes. Several hundred cases of blindness due to these worms have been reported in children from around the world in the past several years.

The symptoms children have depend on the number of eggs they've swallowed and on which organs of their body have been invaded. Many children have no symptoms, others a fever and swelling of the liver and a few pneumonia, pains in muscles and joints and trouble with their vision. Medical experts have given this disease the name *Visceral Larva Migrans,* which in Latin roughly means, "young worms migrating through the organs." In an attempt to control this infection, Todd and Latimer came up with an excellent proposal.

"We'll require that all dogs and cats sold in pet shops or transferred from one owner to another be dewormed beforehand," Todd had told me several weeks before.

"You won't be able to enforce it among private owners," I warned him.

"But I can see to it that the pet shops comply, and that's better than nothing," he said.

I fully supported the proposal. At last we would be doing something about controlling *Toxocara* infections! Within a few weeks, it became part of the Health Code.

"What is Latimer saying at the City Council?" I asked Todd.

"That we don't think the bill is a good idea as it's presently written."

"Fine." I replied. "We would be responsible for enforcing it and we just don't have the manpower for that."

"And you can be sure," Todd interjected, "that the City Fathers aren't going to give us any additional manpower."

What Todd and I didn't know at the time was how successful voluntary compliance would be on the part of dog owners. It would have been an impossible task for our meager staff to hand out summonses to dog owners violating the law in addition to inspecting 30,000 restaurants and eating places, controlling rats, inspecting the water supply and sewers and seeing that milk was properly dated. When a law was finally passed several years later, with enforcement spread out among several city departments, I was surprised to see how many dog owners complied. But compliance was better in Manhattan and areas where looks and comments from neighbors prodded people into obeying the law. But in the outlying boroughs dogs still defecated in the parks.

When Latimer returned he said, "Can I tell you what happened down at City Hall?"

"Yes, what did happen?"

"The usual."

"I haven't been here long enough to know what the usual is. You'll have to tell me."

"The Women's League for the Protection of Children from Dogs and Other Animal Nuisances was represented by Mrs. Gerta Spritz, the president. She did her usual thing, saying that dogs should be outlawed in the city. As she spoke, someone from the

184

Midtown Humane Society booed and threw some dog feces at her."

"They did that at the hearing?"

"That's right. Oh, they've done it before, many times before. Why, I've been at some meetings where they've thrown the stuff all over the place."

"Then what happened?"

"The chairman had the dog-poop thrower ejected and Mrs. Spritz continued talking."

"Was anything definitive decided about the new law?"

"No, and my guess is that it will take several years for the measure to pass the Council."

As it turned out Latimer was right. The measure wasn't passed into law by the City Council until 1978.

CHAPTER 15

PERIL ON THE BEACH

As spring turned into summer, I completed my first six months as Director of the Bureau. I was learning that the city's bureaucracy was complex and ponderous, an incredible red-tape factory where new ideas were immobilized until they died. New ideas weren't crippled within the Health Department, but by the maze of checks and balances on it from other branches of city government. The Commissioner of Health and his top staff liked my plans for replacing the part-time physicians with nurse epidemiologists. But an incredible series of obstacles lay ahead.

The concept was straightforward and simple. Ten public-health nurses presently working for the department and with ten years of experience would be taken into the program. They would be given a three-month didactic course in a medical center and taught epidemiology, biostatistics, public-health administration, microbiology and environmental sanitation. The course would cost the department fifty thousand dollars. After completing it they would train for nine months in the field under my supervision and that of the five best part-time physician epidemiologists I planned to keep.

Since the nurses were already on the city payroll, the cost in salaries consisted only of a two-thousand-dollar raise apiece as compensation for their increased skills. The majority of the part-time physician epidemiologists would be terminated, representing a saving of $450,000 per year. Not only would the city save that much money per year, but also it would have ten well-trained full-time epidemiologists on board.

My seemingly simple plan had to move through six separate but related bureaucracies and within each of these there was layer upon layer of internal checks and balances. At first I was impatient with this tedious swamp of bureaucratic process. I suspected that maybe the Commissioner and his top staff were saying yes to me while killing the plan behind the scenes. After all, the Commissioner was in a powerful position. He could cut through all of the red tape overnight if he really wanted to. How wrong I was. But I only learned that when I became Commissioner of Health myself four and a half years later.

With time I became more tolerant of red tape. I had no other choice. But I also learned that the system wasn't unbeatable. It was vulnerable to two weapons—tenacity and endurance. And I made every effort to develop both.

The passage of six months also witnessed twelve pay periods for which I never received a check.

"We can arrange a loan from the Commissioner's Fund," Murray said when I complained, mistakingly blaming him. "And it ain't me, Doctor. I swear to that. It's that damn Budget Bureau."

"Why should it take so long?"

"They're just slow, that's all. And they keep your money, invest it and make interest on it. Then when they pay you, you don't get the interest, just the money."

"That's unethical." I was indignant.

"Nothing you can do about it. Been doing it for years."

Fortunately, I was living with my brother Gerard at the time and he was practicing law. So I wasn't in dire straights. But suppose I had a family to support? "You'd be in trouble," Bill Herbert said. "Thank God I get paid by the Federal Government."

When I finally did get paid, it was at a lower salary than agreed on. "That's because we're getting a pay hike next month. Once it comes through your salary will be up to what it's supposed to be." That was the long and short of Murray's explanation. So not only were they holding back my money and using it to generate interest income for the city, but they were also shortchanging me to boot.

And in spite of tricks like this, the city was still drifting toward bankruptcy.

During the six months, I had also developed a few insights about which disease reports were important and which weren't. Over two hundred calls came into the office each week, from physicians, hospitals, private citizens and clinics, reporting different problems. And then there were the yellow "395" report cards which flowed in every day, reporting everything from hepatitis to chickenpox. The bureau was like a massive triage station. Everyone had to be alert, on his toes, to pick up on the reports which were significant. Not an easy job. Bill Herbert and I had to scan the reports each day to see if there were any epidemic patterns emerging. Private physicians might report cases of hepatitis in individual patients. But only we could see if there was a pattern to them. Sometimes there was. A dozen individual doctors in a given part of the city might each report a case apiece. That meant to us that there was clustering—a grouping of cases in a small geographic area. It pointed the finger to a common source of infection which we would have to find to prevent the disease from spreading.

But we knew that there were many such clustered outbreaks which escaped us. People might all be exposed in a restaurant, go to their private physicians in distant parts of the city or out in the suburbs and we'd never be the wiser. It was when people who knew each other got sick from a common source that we would see a lead. Invariably one of the reporting physicians would tell us, "His friends have the same problem too."

Frequently, doctors called and reported what they thought was a rare, serious disease. "I think it's smallpox," one doctor said to me over the phone one day. "And the lady just got back from India."

I rushed out to his office to investigate. There was still a lot of smallpox in India. The woman had been vaccinated two years before. But Indian smallpox was extremely virulent and severe. It was well known among experts that a vaccination more than a year old didn't give much protection against the disease in many people. When I saw the woman there was no doubt. She had an allergic rash.

"I'm terribly sorry for making you come out here like that," the physician said.

189

"Don't be sorry," I told him. "I'd rather have false alarms than bad surprises."

A steady rush of false alarms together with a constant flow of reports about simple and unimportant communicable diseases can blurr the eagle-eyed vision a medical detective must maintain all the time. I came to recognize this during my first six months in New York City. It wasn't Africa, where massive epidemics came roaring up a river valley or swept through an entire city. That era in the history of communicable diseases ended in the United States in the early part of the century. Vaccines, improved sanitation and hygiene and high standards of living relegated most killing communicable disease epidemics to the shelves of history. Maybe the epidemics are shelved, but the diseases aren't. They are still here, lying in wait, so to speak, and while they may not cause large epidemics, they are capable of spreading to a sizable number of people and taking lives.

All of this meant I had to readjust my sights, refine my instincts, polish my analytic skills and look at everything with a jeweler's eyepiece and not with my bare eyes as I did in Africa. The killers are more sinister here than in Africa and Asia. They lurk unseen and then when least expected strike by surprise. I learned to take nothing at face value, to question everything, to follow up on every lead, however absurd. I was glad I did.

Murray and Ida Peters came into my office almost every day with a lead that needed running down. One day Ida came in and said, "A Dr. Mancuso called from Brooklyn. He has a problem he wants to discuss with you."

"What is it?"

"He wouldn't say. I asked him. He wants to talk to you and to you alone."

I called Dr. Mancuso right away.

"Dr. Imperato," he started off, "maybe you can help me with something. I had a patient in Sackett Hospital, a ten-year-old-boy, who died a few hours ago. Peculiar case. His name was Tommy Madison."

"Ten years, is that what you said?" I made notes on a pad of yellow legal paper.

"Yes. His mother called me just a week ago. Said he had the flu. You know, fever, body aches, the whole bit."

"Did he have a sore throat?"

"No."

"Runny nose?"

"No."

"How high was the fever?"

"Started off at 102 or so and then went up to 106."

"One hundred and six! That's damn high."

"Yes, I know. That's why I had them bring him into the hospital three days later. He wasn't getting any better on aspirin."

"Was anyone else in the family sick?"

"That's what I'm coming to. You see, when I got this boy into the hospital he had a funny rash. Looked like measles. But his mother said he had them already."

"Where did it start? Do you know that?"

"I didn't see it start. But his mother says it started on his ankles and wrists and then moved up until it got to his forehead. By the time I saw him it was all over."

"Looked like measles, you say?" I was writing it all down.

"Yes, just like it, but a little different."

"What was different about it?"

"Well some of the spots looked like they had blood in them."

"Uh, huh. Did he have a rash inside his mouth?"

There was a pause. "Come to think of it, yes, he did."

"How about on the soles of his feet and his palms?"

"Yes, he had that too. That's why I made a diagnosis of Coxsackie virus infection."

"What made you think that?"

"The rash, fever and the fact that he didn't respond to high doses of penicillin. The fever just stayed up there at 106 until he died. Had to be a virus. You know penicillin doesn't touch them."

"You said before that someone else in the family had the same illness."

"Yes, his seven-year-old brother Eddie. He came down with it three days after Tommy and I hospitalized him too."

"Have you treated him the same way?"

"Yes, penicillin, aspirin and bed rest."

"What is his condition now?"

"Not good. He's going the same way as his brother. This virus is virulent. Got all the nurses in the hospital upset. Afraid they're going to catch it."

"Have you done any blood tests yet?"

191

"Just the routine ones."

"How about antibody studies?"

"To tell you the truth, no. I didn't. I just don't know what to do next and that's why I called you."

"I have a couple of quick questions. Were these children out of the city at all in the past few weeks?"

"As a matter of fact, they were. They went out to the Hamptons to visit their uncle for a couple of days. He has a house there."

"When were they out there?"

"About a week before Tommy got sick."

"Did they go down to the beach?"

"I'm not sure, but I can find out."

"Where is Eddie now?"

"Room 225."

"O.K." I said, "find out whatever you can. And then can you meet me at the hospital in an hour?"

"Absolutely."

I called Herbert and Latimer and they came on the double. I gave them a rundown on the two cases.

"Two children with a febrile infection and a macular rash with petechiae. Doesn't respond to penicillin. The rash started on the ankles and wrists and spread to the trunk and head. They both gave a history of having been out in the Hamptons a week before the illness started in Tommy."

"Did they walk around on the beach or through weeds?" Latimer asked.

"He didn't know, but I suspect they did."

They both looked at me. "You know what I'm thinking of, don't you?" I asked.

"Sure do," Bill replied.

"Let's go then. Dr. Latimer, do you have your instruments?"

"Right here." He raised the small leather bag for me to see."

Sackett Hospital was a small private institution, a modern plant with pretty rooms and creature comforts like TV in every room, drapes around the windows and menus which were as good as those in the best restaurants. We quickly found Eddie in Room 225. Dr. Mancuso was already there.

He was a handsome little boy with black hair and blue eyes who broke a smile for us even though he had a fever of 105. Get-well cards stood on the bureau and the night stand. He didn't know that Tommy was dead.

"We told him he had to be taken to another part of the hospital for tests," Dr. Mancuso whispered.

In spite of his ordeal, Eddie gave us a good history. He and Tommy had spent many hours along the beaches, walking through the weeds.

"Did you get bitten by anything, a bug of any kind?" I asked.

He nodded no.

"Nothing bit you. You're sure of that?"

He was sure.

"Probably didn't feel it," Latimer said. "One usually doesn't."

"Did you walk through any weeds here in the city?"

He nodded no.

Bill and I then examined him. He was covered from head to foot with a spotty rash. The spots were red and flat, known as macules in medical language.

"What do you think?" Dr. Mancuso whispered in my ear. "A virus, right?"

I motioned him out into the corridor. Latimer said he wanted to stay behind and go through Eddie's hair.

"Well, what do you think?" Mancuso asked anxiously.

"Rocky Mountain spotted fever."

"What?" he gasped. "Impossible! They only have that out West."

"Not so," Bill said. "Most of it is right here in the East."

"Well I'll be—then why's it called Rocky Mountain spotted fever? Why not Long Island fever?"

"Because that's where it was first discovered and described," Bill replied.

"Mosquito?"

"No, a tick," I replied. "It's carried by ticks."

"Will we get it?" Dr. Mancuso asked in a hushed voice.

"No, don't worry. It's not spread from man to man, only from ticks to man."

Neither Bill nor I expected Dr. Mancuso to be familiar with Rocky Mountain spotted fever. He, like most physicians, had been trained to think of the common diseases first, the horses. And he had done that and come up with a plausible diagnosis of a Coxsack-

193

ie virus infection. But Bill and I had been trained to think of the unusual, the zebras, and this disease was one of them. Mancuso had shown sound judgment in contacting us. He realized that he was dealing with something unusual and apparently he wasn't comfortable any longer with his own diagnosis. It didn't kill children this way.

"We've got to get tetracycline going right away," I told him. "Start with a loading dose of 3 grams and then give a gram four times a day."

He rushed over to the nurses' station and came running back with the antibiotic that would wipe out the microbe that had killed Eddie's brother.

"Dr. Imperato! Dr. Herbert!" Latimer called from Eddie's room. We rushed in. "I've found one here on the back of his head." I bent over to look. Sure enough, there it was, a large tick bloated up with blood.

"*Dermacentor variabilis,*" Latimer said.

"What?" Mancuso grimaced.

"The dog tick," Latimer continued. It's the commonest species in this part of the United States."

Latimer removed the tick, a delicate job, but one he knew how to do well. "Now, that didn't hurt, did it?" he said to Eddie. He put the tick into a dry sterile jar. Then all of us walked out of the room.

"I'll take it up to the laboratory and I'm sure we'll grow out *Rickettsia rickettsii.*"

"Is that the name of the bacteria?" Mancuso asked.

"It's not a bacterium," Latimer replied. "It's a rickettsia. They're sort of midway between viruses and bacteria. These rickettsia are hardy organisms, can be passed by the mother tick to her eggs. When the eggs hatch and the offspring grow up they carry the rickettsia in their bodies. Then they bite someone and the bites are often painless. They burrow their heads into the skin and salivate as they drink the person's blood. The rickettsia are passed into the person with the tick's saliva. Then when the tick has had enough, it drops off."

"How often do they bite people?" Mancuso asked.

Latimer tightened the lid of the jar where he had put the tick. "They can go for a couple of months without a blood meal if they've had a good one to start."

194

Eddie improved dramatically over the next few days and finally recovered. We contacted his family and got a list of all those who had been in the same areas with him and Tommy and then we contacted all of these people. None of them had been bitten by ticks and none of them contracted the disease. But to be on the safe side, we placed them under surveillance and gave them preventive doses of tetracycline. Bill sent all of our findings to the Suffolk County Health Department, which possesses great expertise on this disease since it deals with several cases each year. The tick Latimer removed from Eddie's head was positive for *Rickettsia rickettsii* and studies on Eddie's blood demonstrated beyond a shadow of a doubt that he had Rocky Mountain spotted fever. Bill and I concluded that Tommy and Eddie had ventured into an area where there were infected ticks, an area where the adults who were with them probably didn't go. They were young boys and could easily have jumped into a patch of tall grass or run through it while the adults walked on the sandy beach a few feet away.

Ticks carrying Rocky Mountain spotted fever are still present in many areas of the United States, along beaches, in weeds, brush and woodlands. Every year, especially during the spring and summer months, a number of cases of the disease occur in areas around New York City. The disease can be severe and fatal, especially if it is not diagnosed and properly treated in time. To help doctors think of this zebra, health departments in the New York metropolitan area send out advisories to them each spring and summer. And local newspapers help by carrying stories alerting people to the possibility of the disease and its association with ticks. The New York City Department of Health collects ticks from all the city's beaches during the spring and examines them for the possible presence of the microbe. None has been found in recent years. But infected ticks have been found on Long Island and in the woodlands to the north of the city. The influx of hundreds of thousands of travelers into these areas each summer increases the chances of the disease occurring. Epidemics will not break out, but there will always be those few who will contract the disease like Tommy and Eddie and perhaps die if they don't receive proper treatment.

CHAPTER 16

A LETHAL SORE THROAT

My first summer in the bureau passed quickly. It was a kaleido-
scope of problems. Bill Herbert and I went through June and July
dealing with a number of epidemics and outbreaks. There was a serious outbreak of staphylococcal skin infections in over seventy in-
fants in a Queens hospital nursery. We investigated it thoroughly
and found that the problem was sloppy nursery technique. No
sooner was the nursery epidemic over than an epidemic of sep-
ticemia broke out in a Brooklyn hospital. We finally tracked down
the source of this blood infection to intravenous solutions which
had been contaminated during the manufacturing and bottling
process. This was followed by three major outbreaks of *salmonella*
food poisoning, an outbreak of aseptic meningitis in a day camp
and a measles outbreak in the Bronx.

Todd and Latimer had their hands full with other problems. An
average of a thousand dog bites were reported every day during the
summer months. It was hot. The dogs were out loose on the streets
and they were irritable. "Dog-children contact," as Todd called it,
was at its peak. Those thousand bites per day generated twice as
many incoming telephone calls to the Veterinary Division and a
deluge of paper work. Todd's four policemen were kept hopping
not only with the dog-bite problem, but with everything from oce-

lots to snakes. By the end of August, Latimer and the policemen chalked up a record which included catching an ocelot which had escaped from its owner on the Fourteenth Street station of the IRT subway in Manhattan, confiscating ten puff adders shipped into Kennedy Airport and searching for a man who sold a four-foot-long copperhead, along with a vial of antivenom to a fourteen-year-old boy in the Bronx Zoo. The boy was bitten by the snake an hour later and rushed to the emergency room of a nearby hospital where he was given the antivenom. He had an allergic reaction to it, but fortunately recovered. Latimer and the policemen spent a lot of their time on snake problems. But they were also deluged with complaints about birds, alligators, monkeys and ocelots. Ocelots were very popular at the time and it really amazed me to see the number of complaints we got about them. But it was the snakes which frightened people most, and which caused me the most concern. Some of the snakes people kept were unusual vipers from Africa for which there was no antivenom in New York City. One bite and a person could be dead. The thought of what might have happened to that fourteen-year-old boy if he hadn't had antivenom haunted me.

August ended that year with a ten-day heat wave. The news was full of stories about brownouts, blackouts, overheated cars, open fire hydrants, falling water pressure and the air-pollution index. The decrepit air conditioner in my office browned out on the third day. But at least there was a faint breeze which blew in from the park below. I felt exhausted not only from the heat but from the constant barrage of problems, big and small, which kept coming in. I now understood why people like Todd and Murray didn't change anything. How could they? They didn't have any energy left at the end of the day to get out of the trap. It was not only a trap created by fifty years of public-health legislation, but also a prison of public demands and expectations. What the public wanted wasn't what they necessarily needed. Changing procedures which people viewed as life-insuring meant reeducating them. It wasn't going to be easy. I knew it now better than before and because I knew it I had greater respect for my staff.

The heat wave had struck the borough of Queens hard. There had been no electricity for several days in some sections and because of the scorching, humid heat many had taken to sleeping out-side on roofs, in backyards and on front lawns. People in Queens always complained about bad sewers, poor transportation and pot-hole-riddled streets. Now they were without electricity.

While I was coping with the steady flow of problems coming into the bureau, a five-year-old girl who lived in Queens came down with a sore throat. Jennifer Krauss had blonde hair and blue eyes. She lived in the Jamaica area of Queens on Centerville Street. It was once the home of prosperous businessmen. But now it was a decaying heap of old wooden clapboard houses, peeling paint, sag-ging porches, weeds and broken pavements. The area had become what is euphemistically called "an inner-city area." People living there had to cope with grinding poverty, social discrimination and disintegration, crime and a sense of hopelessness. It was a pre-dominantly black area, but there were some white families living there because like the blacks they were on welfare.

Jennifer was one of fifteen children. Her father, John Krauss, worked in a factory, but his salary was scarcely enough to keep the family afloat. His wife, Gilda, did the best she could to stretch ev-ery dollar. But even with stretching she couldn't make ends meet. The Krausses were on welfare because of this and the Department of Social Services sent them a monthly stipend check and paid their rent. The free rent was a mixed blessing because they had to live wherever the Department of Social Services found them a place. The Krausses weren't viewed as an asset by landlords in middle-class neighborhoods. They ended up in slum areas where short leases enabled landlords to hike the rent at frequent intervals. It got hiked above what the Department of Social Services was willing to pay and this meant that the Krausses had to move almost every year. Jennifer had already lived in four places and now there was talk they would have to move again. She had heard the land-lord tell her father that he could rent his six-room wooden house to two families and double the rent income. She didn't know what it all meant except that they would have to move again.

When Jennifer first complained of a sore throat, her mother didn't make much of it. After all, Jennifer and her brothers and sis-ters had just recovered from the measles. And before that they had all had chickenpox. She felt Jennifer's forehead, then her own.

199

There wasn't any difference. But later in the day, Jennifer complained of feeling very tired. Gilda Krauss thought it was the heat. The heat made everyone feel tired.

She didn't make any connection between Jennifer's sore throat and the one six-year-old Betty had three months before. Betty had become very ill and Gilda and her husband had taken her to the emergency room of a small nearby hospital. The doctor on duty said it was just a sore throat and he gave Betty a shot of some kind. But once home, Betty got worse. Gilda and John Krauss took her back to the emergency room, where she died a few minutes after the same doctor examined her again. "It's rare, but it happens," he told them. Betty died of a bad sore throat and that was that.

Jennifer coughed all night long and when she got up in the morning Gilda noticed that her neck was swollen. She thought it was probably swollen glands, which went along with a lot of sore throats. But by noon, Jennifer had trouble swallowing and Gilda figured she had better take her to the hospital. She went to the same emergency room where she had taken Betty back in May.

There was a lot of hectic activity in my office that same morning. We received a call from the Center for Disease Control that the Quarantine Service had delayed the docking of an oil tanker because of a suspected case of smallpox on board. The captain of the ship had telephoned ahead saying that one of his crewmen, Ali Midda, a native of West Bengal, India, was down with a rash. There was a lot of smallpox in West Bengal at the time so we had to take the report very seriously. I sent Bill Herbert out to the ship to investigate. He got there by driving to Staten Island where the U.S. Public Health Service quarantine cutter took him out to the ship which was anchored near the Chevron Oil Docks in Perth Amboy, New Jersey. The patient was frightened out of his wits, Bill later reported. He found out that Ali Midda left West Bengal on August 15 with thirty-two other Indians and flew to Baltimore where they joined twelve Italians as the crew of the American freighter. Three days later the ship sailed for Venezuela and then came to New York. Bill was pretty sure it was chickenpox because of the kind of rash, its distribution on Ali Midda's body and because Ali Midda had several recent vaccinations against smallpox, including one early in the month. But he took no chances. A temporary quarantine was placed on the ship and its crew until the CDC could examine the specimens Bill obtained from Ali Midda's rash.

"It's a wild thing," he said when he came back. "You know what these Americans shippers do? They fly these Indians in here and board them on ships right under our noses. It's cheaper for them to do it this way than to hire Americans. "It's a flying merchant marine. Wild!"

"Maybe it's a flying merchant marine," I said, "but you're going to become a flying epidemiologist."

"What?"

"CDC isn't taking any chances on this one. They want the specimens hand-carried down there right away."

Bill flew off to Atlanta on the next plane while Ali Midda and his fellow flying crewmen were grounded on the ship. The hot, muggy afternoon wore on. I looked down on Foley Square through the open window. People were poking their way along the hot pavements almost aimlessly as if devoid of energy and purpose. The ice-cream and soft-drink vendors were doing a booming trade on the corners and some young men sat on the edge of the pool fountain in Federal Plaza with their mod trousers rolled up and their bare feet in the water. The sycamore trees stood still. Not a leaf fluttered. And beyond them, down the canyon which was Nassau Street, the Wall Street skyscrapers stood shrouded in thick layers of polluted air.

As Bill was flying off to Atlanta, Georgia, Jennifer Krauss was being examined in the emergency room where her sister had died. There was another doctor on duty and he told Gilda he didn't know what Jennifer had. He recommended she be transferred by ambulance to Central Queens Hospital. It was a much larger institution, he told Gilda, and one with better facilities for diagnosing and treating Jennifer.

The phone rang and jolted my listless gazing down on the square. Ida Peters picked it up. Parts of her conversation drifted over to me with the droning of the old wall fan behind her desk. I could only hear parts of it.

"Five years old, you say . . . extremely . . . what . . . oh . . . transfer . . . of course there could be an epidemic . . . yes, he is . . . right away . . ."

201

She put the phone down and came running over to my desk. The look on her face told me it was something serious. "Bad problem, Ida?"

"Sounds like it, Doctor. It's a Dr. Elizabeth Holmes from the emergency room of Central Queens Hospital. She's the pediatric resident on duty and has a very sick child there."

I picked up the phone. "My name is Elizabeth Holmes," said the voice on the other end. "We just received a five-year-old girl on transfer from the Sutphin Infirmary. She's in very bad shape."

"What's the problem?"

"Five-day history of sore throat, neck swelling and severe cough."

"Is it streptococcal?"

"Er, I don't think so. Her temp is 102, her respirations 36 a minute and labored, pulse 124 and blood pressure 90 over 60.

As she spoke, my mind ran down the list of possibilities. If it wasn't a strep throat then it was a rare bird . . . or rather, a zebra. And what raced through my mind was Vincent's angina, rhinovirus infection, fungus infections, infectious mononucleosis and diphtheria.

"What did you find in her throat?"

Holmes replied that Jennifer's throat was covered with a dirty white membrane. As far as I was concerned that ruled out the fungus infections, rhinovirus infection and Vincent's angina, leaving infectious mono, a strep throat and diphtheria.

"Is her palate paralyzed?" Holmes said it wasn't. If Jennifer had diphtheria there was a fifty-fifty chance her palate would be paralyzed. "How about the electrocardiogram?"

"Shows S-T depression in leads I, II and AVF."

"So she's got myocardial damage. That's an important finding."

Jennifer's clinical findings pointed to a diagnosis of diphtheria. But the epidemiologic evidence stood strongly against it. In the previous five years in New York City there had been only two cases. The disease was rarer than a zebra even in New York where everything is said to be found. In the early 1900s there were about 15,000 cases a year in the city. But this pattern changed in 1928 when diphtheria toxoid became available and mass-vaccination campaigns were begun. By 1930 there were only 3,000 cases a year and by 1946 only 386 cases. The curve kept falling, 72 cases in 1950 and 4 cases in 1960.

If Jennifer had diphtheria where on earth did she get it? I had to make some fast decisions. Time was of the essence. If it was diphtheria every minute counted for Jennifer. Every minute witnessed the production of thousands of molecules of a powerful toxin by the diphtheria microbes. They would circulate through the bloodstream and find their targets, the nerve and heart muscle cells. And they would destroy them. Antibiotics could kill off the microbes and that would stop the production of toxin. But they would have no effect on the toxin already in Jennifer's body. Only large doses of diphtheria antitoxin could neutralize it. Without it, nerve and heart muscle cells would die every minute, and if too many died so would Jennifer.

If it was diphtheria, I had to find out where Jennifer got it from. And I had to find it out fast. Others might be picking it up from the same source. And they and Jennifer might have spread it to others in turn. This is how epidemics and outbreaks are born. I had to get out there and track down everyone who had contact with Jennifer and this had to be done immediately.

I reflected as Dr. Holmes spoke. I weighed everything in a couple of seconds and made a decision. "Treat her as a case of diphtheria. Start the antibiotics and the antitoxin immediately."

The epidemiologist uses the laboratory to sort out his suspicions. There are many tests which can be used to confirm or rule out a diagnosis and one group of these is based on the principle of identifying the microbe. This is done by taking a specimen of infectious material from the patient and putting it into substances which it thrives on. The diphtheria microbe is very fond of a broth which is made from beef serum and whole egg, a concoction known as Loeffler's medium, named after the microbiologist who first developed it in the late nineteenth century. When a sample of the diphtheria microbe is placed on a sterile mix of Loeffler's medium, it grows and multiplies by leaps and bounds. Within a matter of hours it can be isolated.

I told Dr. Holmes to send samples from Jennifer's throat to Dr. Eleanor Williams at the Health Department Bureau of Laboratories on First Avenue and 27th Street. "Have them hand-carried over there right away. If it's diphtheria we'll know it within a matter of twenty-four hours." To complete the workup, other samples had to be run through the laboratory to rule out fungus infections, infectious mono, streptococci and other bacteria which might mimic diphtheria. My guess was that they would all be negative. But I couldn't be absolutely sure. In this business the expected wasn't always found, and, alas, the unexpected turned up with alarming frequency.

The isolation unit at Central Queens Hospital was a large suite of rooms. Over the swinging door entrance was a large sign in bold black lettering: Do Not Enter—Authorized Personnel Only. Jennifer was put in a room to herself on a spotlessly clean bed with shiny aluminum side rails. A large quart bottle of intravenous fluid dangled from a pole at the head of the bed. The black print on the blue and white label read "Normal Saline Solution," a salt and water mix in the same proportions usually found in the tissues of the body. Dr. Holmes had inserted six million units of penicillin into the bottle and scribbled this fact on the label with a black felt-tipped pen. The drops fell quickly out of the bottle and into a cylinderlike reservoir and then down the plastic tubing into Jennifer's bloodstream. Each drop carried salt, water and penicillin molecules. The penicillin traveled throughout her body and to the blood vessels lining the wall of her throat. They went into prompt action, helping the white blood cells which had been there trying to kill off the invading microbes.

Penicillin is effective not only against the diphtheria organism but also against a number of other bacteria which we hadn't ruled out. No matter how one looked at it, we had everything to gain and nothing to lose by using it. But diphtheria antitoxin was the only thing that was going to save Jennifer from the damaging effects of the toxin which I suspected was destroying her vital organs. It's a clear yellow fluid made from horse serum. Some people are allergic to it and Dr. Holmes and I had no way of knowing how Jennifer would react when it was injected. But it was a risk we had to take. Dr. Holmes injected 50,000 units of the antitoxin into the intravenous tubing and another into the muscles of Jennifer's right buttocks. A massive dose. But it wasn't too small in a situation like this where vital cells were dying every fraction of a second. Jennifer tolerated it well.

Jennifer's brothers and sisters and her playmates on Centerville Street were vulnerable. She had shared candy and ice cream with them and had coughed in their faces. I had to start a dragnet of all the kids on the block and find out if they were immunized against diphtheria. The same thing had to be done with all of the members of the Krauss family. Throat cultures had to be taken on all of them. And one culture wasn't enough. I knew we would have to take several on successive days to turn up the diphtheria microbe if it was there.

I couldn't do this myself and Bill Herbert was still in Atlanta and wouldn't be back until the following day. He had called soon after I had finished talking to Dr. Holmes to say that the specimens from Ali Midda, the Indian seaman, were positive for chickenpox. So the quarantine on the ship was lifted and it pulled into its berth. Bill had never seen diphtheria and wanted to get involved in the investigation. But I couldn't wait until morning.

There was only one solution. The nurses. They could do it. I was sure they could. I called Catherine O'Leary, the public-health nurse in charge of Queens, and told her the story. "I know it's late," I said apologetically, "and I hate to ask you to do this at night and . . ." She cut me short. "No apologies needed. It's got to be done and that's all. No ifs or buts about it. Four of my girls and I are on our way."

Catherine had been a public-health nurse for over twenty years. Her first beat had been the Red Hook section of Brooklyn, then known as a "tough neighborhood" in an era before neighborhoods became "dangerous." That was a time when a doctor's white coat and black bag and a blue public-health nurse's uniform commanded respect and insured safety in a rough neighborhood. Times had changed.

By the time I got to the Krauss house after a subway, elevated train and bus ride, Catherine had been at work for almost two hours. She was seated on the edge of a bed in the living room talking with Gilda Krauss, a petite woman now drawn and pale. Catherine had already collected a list of forty-seven contacts. Twenty-two of them were of school age. "I'll be able to check out the school immunizations on the twenty-two tomorrow morning," she said. "With the others it's hard to say. Catch as catch can."

Gilda Krauss told us that none of them were immunized against anything as far as she knew. "Didn't the children ever get immunized in school?" I asked her. She didn't think so because they were moved around so much and never stayed in a school long enough for the immunization teams to reach them. "They just slipped through the net," Catherine said. "It happens in instances like this."

Catherine's four nurses were up and down the block getting the first throat cultures on the forty-seven contacts. She had already taken cultures on all of the Krauss children, most of whom were out with the nurses on the street. "They look okay, but I'm suspicious about David, age nine, and John, age two. They have sore throats. They slept in the same room with Jennifer."

My examination of David and John confirmed Catherine's impression. I strongly suspected they had diphtheria and sent them to Central Queens Hospital, where they were admitted to the isolation unit by Dr. Holmes. But everyone else in the family was well and had no signs of sore throats.

Catherine and her nurses had gone out with diphtheria toxoid and bottles of erythromycin. We gave a shot of toxoid to all of the members of the Krauss family and to the neighborhood contacts. This would start the development of antibodies in those who didn't have any and build up the levels in those who had some already. A second shot would be given in a month to those who had no record of previous immunizations and this would be followed by a third shot in a year. We gave erythromycin to all of the members of the family and to the forty-seven contacts on the block. It's an antibiotic which quickly kills off the diphtheria microbe. I knew this would adversely affect our subsequent throat cultures. By the time we took them, the organism would be wiped out by the erythromycin in most but not all instances where it was now present. But I had to put the welfare of these people ahead of my strong desires as a medical detective to pinpoint the source and chart the chain of spread.

Early the next morning, the laboratories called with the report. "It's definitely *Corynebacterium diphtheriae*," said Dr. Williams. My hunch was right. It was the diphtheria microbe. I called Dr. Holmes and gave her the news. "It's what we suspected," she replied somewhat sorrowfully. Jennifer wasn't doing well in spite of

206

the fact that the infection was being quickly brought under control. "She still has S-T depressions and I'm worried by all of those extra heartbeats she's having. I just don't know what more I can do."

"You've done all you can," I told her. "The toxin has had a five-day lead on us. It's been destroying Jennifer's myocardium. We can't reverse that. We're not God."

My words didn't comfort Dr. Holmes. I could tell by the way she responded. But there was nothing we could do to reverse the damage already done to Jennifer's heart. Our only hope was that it wasn't so severe as to kill her. The diphtheria toxin mutilates the heart cells to such a degree that the normal electrical impulses which trigger the heartbeat are short-circuited. When these short circuits happen the heart beats irregularly. It would be two to four weeks before we would really know if Jennifer was going to make it or not. And it would take that long for the penicillin to kill off all the microbes layered in the membrane in her throat. As long as those microbes lived they produced toxin. The antitoxin we had given Jennifer would continue to circulate throughout her body and each molecule of it would link up with a molecule of toxin and neutralize it. The membrane in Jennifer's throat wasn't large enough to cause problems with her breathing. It's not a problem in most cases and contrary to popular belief people with diphtheria don't generally die from suffocation because of the membrane, but because of heart failure and cardiac arrest.

The following day Dr. Williams called from the laboratory to say that the throat cultures were positive on four other Krauss children in addition to David and John. I sent all the children to Dr. Holmes and she started them on treatment with antitoxin and antibiotics as she had with David and John. These four children were perfectly healthy. They didn't even have sore throats. It pointed out how variable this diphtheria microbe is in how it affects people. And it made me suspect that the microbe had probably moved through the family from person to person and only caused visible illness in Betty, Jennifer, David and John.

None of the forty-seven neighborhood contacts were positive, which was a great relief. I telephoned Dr. Holmes to bring her up to date on some of the details of the laboratory tests which were still going on. "David and John are doing fine," she said. "No reactions to the antitoxin. I was really worried about that. And the other four have tolerated the antitoxin just as well. They'll be all right."

Jennifer was still holding her own and we both had raised hopes of her coming through without too much permanent damage to her heart. We talked a lot about that over the phone, just how much cardiac damage Jennifer would have.

We continued our investigation that day with ever-growing intensity. I checked with the chief medical examiner about Betty. I was almost sure she died from diphtheria in May. An autopsy had been performed at the hospital where she died, but no signs of the disease were found. That didn't exclude it though. If a pathologist weren't looking for it he might miss it, especially in the early stages. Would exhuming the body and reexamining it help? No, because all traces of the disease would be gone from the remains. Betty's death had been listed as "severe pharyngitis" on her death certificate.

"Then where did she get it?" Bill asked. I didn't know. Somehow the bacillus got into the Krauss family. This could have happened through a healthy carrier. The germ is always around, but because most people have been immunized against it, it doesn't manifest its presence by causing disease. It moves around unnoticed and causes no harm. "You and I could be carriers from time to time," I told Bill. "We wouldn't even know the thing was in our throats."

But the Krauss family was a fertile field for this microbe because they were devoid of any antibody defenses. I suspected that the germ had gotten in sometime in May and slowly moved through the family. There was little point in trying to demonstrate how it got into the household. So ubiquitous a microbe could have come in with almost anyone.

Gilda Krauss went to visit her children in the isolation unit the following morning. After spending a few minutes with the six healthy children she went down the hall to Jennifer's room. She spoke to her for a while telling her that she would be able to come home soon. Dr. Holmes passed by in the corridor and Gilda went out to speak with her. "She's holding her own, Mrs. Krauss, but it's hard to say at this point. She's still a very sick little girl."

Gilda went back into Jennifer's room and stood by her bedside.

Jennifer told her mother she needed to urinate. Gilda asked a nurse to bring in a bedpan. The nurse put it under Jennifer and just as she turned to leave the bedside, a pale hue flashed over Jennifer's face. She was hardly breathing. The nurse pressed the button which sounded a yellow alert.

Dr. Holmes and her staff ran into the room.

"Ventricular fibrillation," she exclaimed, looking up at the TV cardiogram monitor. The electrical impulses controlling Jennifer's heartbeat had short-circuited. Gilda Krauss moved to a corner of the room and clenched her hands. She didn't know what ventricular fibrillation was. But to her Jennifer looked dead. She had the same color Betty had when she died. Dr. Holmes applied the defibrillator to Jennifer's chest. If it worked it would jolt the uncoordinated vibrations of Jennifer's heart back into normal rhythmic beats.

"No effect," the intern said, looking up at the screen. Dr. Holmes tried again and again and each time there was no effect. Gilda's eyes darted from the screen to Jennifer to Dr. Holmes and then the whole image was blurred with tears. Finally, after several minutes, Dr. Holmes gave up. Jennifer was dead.

CHAPTER 17

TOURIST FEVER

I was never able to demonstrate the source of the diphtheria outbreak on Centerville Street. In a sense it didn't have to be demonstrated because it was overshadowed by the far more important piece of knowledge that the diphtheria bacillus is always around. It is in our midst and strikes whenever circumstances bring it into contact with a vulnerable person. The microbe doesn't cause large epidemics in places like New York, Chicago, Los Angeles and other urban areas of the United States, but rather isolated cases which are often deadly. In 1977, the disease struck again in New York City, this time in a family living on the Upper West Side of Manhattan. Two children died. None of the children in this particular family had ever been immunized even though they lived in the shadows of one of the largest medical centers of the world.

The six Krauss children were eventually discharged from Central Queens Hospital. Catherine went to their home to check on their progress and to give emotional support to the family. Gilda Krauss had suffered a hard blow—the loss of two children within a period of three months. But she was grateful for what we and the doctors at the hospital had done for her and her family.

Catherine and her nurses had empirically demonstrated what I firmly believed in, that public-health nurses could function as epidemiologists. The diphtheria outbreak in Queens had been a perfect laboratory in which to test the ability of nurses to function this way.

As fall approached, we geared up for our annual immunization program. Its goal was to get children immunized against all the common communicable diseases. Free immunizations were given out all year long at seventy-eight child-health centers and twenty district-health centers. And the department gave out free vaccine to private physicians to immunize their patients. But in spite of this, almost 30 percent of the children coming into school for the first time lacked all or most of the required immunizations. The bureau's immunization program employed a staff of over thirty people who along with the public-health nurses went through the schools and within six months immunized all the children who needed it. It was protection better late than never. But it didn't solve the problem of preschoolers who weren't immunized, who were vulnerable like Jennifer Krauss to diseases such as diphtheria.

We held health fairs, street-corner immunization clinics, sent community liaison workers knocking on doors and made announcements over radio and on television. But in spite of all this, there was a hard core of complacent parents who didn't bother to have their children immunized because they thought of diseases like diphtheria as a thing of the past. That complacency is still with us. Not even newspaper headlines and TV and radio news reports about children dying of diphtheria, tetanus or polio move complacent parents. For them it's far away, happening to somebody else. They think it will never happen to them or their children. Until it finally does.

The steady flow of exciting challenges which I encountered as New York's chief medical detective brought me into contact with many professional colleagues and before long I felt at home. More and more, Africa receded into the background, although not entirely. My African staff wrote me at unpredictable intervals to send me their good wishes, to tell me they were well and sometimes to ask for things I clearly couldn't send. Some of my former staff didn't think twice about asking me to send a truck, several rifles, a couple of taxicabs, stereo equipment and medicines of all kinds. My replies were always benign and vague and as is their custom I never

212

refused their requests. I simply didn't respond to them and in so doing saved them from the embarrassment a refusal would have caused.

In the early part of 1972, Dr. George Reader, professor and chairman of the Department of Public Health at Cornell University Medical College in New York City, invited me to join the faculty of the school and the staff of New York Hospital. I gladly accepted and was appointed to non-paying positions in both the Department of Public Health and the Department of Medicine. My work at Cornell gave balance to my perspective because it brought me into contact with the ordinary medical problems most patients have. It was also a great intellectual challenge to encounter medical students, not only to teach them but also to learn from them. I spent a half day a week at the Cornell–New York Hospital complex caring for patients in the medical clinic, teaching clinical medicine to the third-year medical students and delivering lectures on public health. My hours there were often interrupted because outbreaks and epidemics aren't respecters of either time or place.

Some of my friends were perplexed by my teaching in a medical school a half day a week since as a city employee I was obviously not working full time. I had to explain to them that Health Department physicians had obtained permission many years ago to spend a half day a week in a teaching center provided the few hours away from the office were offset by overtime. Since we weren't paid for overtime which in most cases was double or triple the half day, the arrangement worked out well. The department also benefited from having members of its staff associated with one of the seven medical schools in the city. And the medical schools were pleased to have the expertise of a public-health official readily available to them.

New York Hospital has one of the finest internal epidemiological services in the country, directed by a physician epidemiologist with a staff of nurse epidemiologists. Dr. Lewis Drusin and I had much in common in terms of our training as internists and public-health experts, and he like myself had also worked in Africa. It was his job to keep an eye out for infections among the thousands of patients who came into the hospital each year. Hospital environments are ideal for the growth and spread of many bacterial infections and hospital patients are highly vulnerable to the complications of

213

these infections, particularly people coming out of surgery, the elderly, the debilitated, the chronically ill and newborn babies.

In 1974, Lew Drusin asked me to assist him in a program which he had developed for sending medical students overseas to developing countries. Some of the students obtained foreign fellowship grants as I had twelve years before, but others took out loans in order to pay for their traveling expenses. I personally arranged programs for students who went to Mali and East Africa. There weren't that many students interested in doing something so unusual as going to Africa, but those who did go were highly motivated and able to adapt to both an alien culture and physical hardship. The letters they wrote back reminded me of those I had written myself several years before. It gave me great pleasure to read of their adventures and exploits, and in their discovery of what was familiar to me, I relived my own past.

It was while I was preparing the fall immunization drive that I received a call from a distraught woman on Staten Island, presenting me with a problem I was able to solve particularly because of my training in tropical medicine and my experience in Africa.

"You must help me, Doctor," she said pleadingly. "My daughter Suzan has been sick with a fever of 104 for the past three days."

"Has she been seen by anyone?"

"Yes, by Dr. Marcus, our family doctor. He said it was the flu and he told me to keep her in bed for a couple of days, to give her aspirin and plenty of fluids."

"Have you followed his advice?"

"Yes," she said, "but she hasn't gotten any better."

"How old is your daughter?"

"Twenty-two."

"What's her occupation?"

"She's a graduate student at New York University."

"Has she been anywhere?"

"Oh, Doctor, you're the first one who has asked me that. I told Dr. Marcus that she had been to Europe for a couple of weeks and that she then took a quick trip to West Africa to visit a friend of hers who works for the State Department and . . ."

I interrupted her. "She was in West Africa?"

"Yes."

214

"Where?"

"Why, Ghana."

"When was she there?"

"Exactly two weeks ago. That is, she left there two weeks ago. But she wasn't there long, just a week, not long enough to pick anything up, I don't think."

"Did you tell Dr. Marcus that Suzan had been to Ghana?"

"I most certainly did. I even said to him that maybe it might be some kind of strange African disease and he told me that I had a fertile imagination."

"Has Suzan had any chills?" I had to move fast. I suspected I was onto something.

"Why, yes, she had terrible chills and she ached all over. That's why Dr. Marcus said she had the flu. I didn't believe him, and called an internal-medicine specialist, a Dr. Murphy, who has an office down the block. He checked her over and said it was the flu. And then you know what he did?"

"No."

"He charged me twenty-five dollars. Can you imagine that? Why, he didn't even examine her very much."

"Did you tell him Suzan had been to Africa?"

"I most certainly did and he said it had nothing to do with her being sick. Have you ever been to Ghana?"

"Yes, I have, a couple of times."

"Thank goodness I've found someone who's been there. You must know what she has."

"Did Suzan take any antimalaria pills before going to Ghana or while she was there?"

"Suzan," I heard her shout, "did you take any pills for malaria? Dr. Imperato of the Health Department wants to know." There was a pause. "What?" Then she said, "No, she didn't. Is there a lot of malaria there?"

"Yes, there is. It's around all the time." I was almost positive that Suzan had malaria. It was nothing to mess around with because the prevailing type in West Africa is caused by a parasite technically known as *Plasmodium falciparum*. This malaria parasite, one of several in the world, causes a malignant form of the disease which is often fatal.

"I can't be absolutely sure," I told Suzan's mother, "but I think she has malaria. I want you to take her to the United States Public Health Service Hospital there on Staten Island right away. I'll call the director and tell him all about Suzan, and that you're on your way."

Suzan and her mother arrived at the hospital fifteen minutes later and a quick blood smear done in the emergency room proved my hunch right.

"It's *P. falciparum*," the director said when he called me back.

Suzan's mother called me on the phone an hour later. "Dr. Imperato, I can't tell you how thankful I am. You saved my Suzan's life. No one else thought of asking if she had been anywhere. All I can say is thank you from the bottom of my heart. You saved my Suzan's life."

Had Suzan gone untreated for another twenty-four hours, chances are she would have lapsed into coma and died. The diagnosis would have been made at autopsy. Almost every year someone dies of malaria in New York City. The story is usually the same. They travel to a malarial area of the world and don't bother to take antimalarial pills to protect themselves. Tourists who travel in groups and on package tours don't often contract the disease because they are warned well in advance by most travel agents about taking health precautions. But many businessmen and some tourists travel solo and don't meet anyone who might suggest the use of antimalarials.

On their return they may develop malaria, which can be fatal. Often the disease manifests itself much like the flu with fever and body aches. Patients may do nothing about it, thinking that it's the flu. An easy-to-cure disease progresses to worse in these individuals, sometimes to the point of no return. They may be hospitalized because of progressive coma and even then the diagnosis may not be made, unless doctors are alert and astute. The malarial deaths which I've seen in New York City have usually taken place when the diagnosis wasn't made soon enough or not at all. What a tragedy it is to see someone die of a perfectly curable disease. A few pills given in time and that's the end of it in most patients.

There are certain strains of *P. falciparum* malaria that are resistant to chloroquine, the drug most often used for preventing and treating the disease. This was a major problem in Vietnam, but it

216

has also cropped up in other parts of the world. The appearance of malaria in someone who has taken chloroquine according to instructions and for the correct period of time raises the possibility that they may have contracted a resistant strain of the parasite. Sporadic cases of this kind have occurred among travelers returning from several areas of the world, including India and Africa. They are rare, however, and most often malaria appears among those who haven't taken a preventive drug or who have taken it improperly.

Suzan might have become the second person to die needlessly of malaria that year. A forty-year-old businessman died two months before in a Manhattan hospital even though the diagnosis was made and treatment started as soon as he hit the emergency room. But he was already in coma and in the third day of his illness. Suzan, however, was luckier. She had a tenacious mother who wasn't satisfied with the advice of two physicians. And she was lucky to come into contact with someone who knew malaria from direct personal experience.

It has never ceased to amaze me how oblivious some travelers are to the dangers of malaria in many parts of the world. Once I was boarding a plane in Dakar, Senegal, for the eight-hour trans-Atlantic flight to New York. It was one in the morning and the plane had already been traveling ten hours, starting in Nairobi and stopping at points along the West African coast. The local manager of the airline, who was a personal friend, came rushing down the aisle to get me a few minutes after I sat down.

"We have a sick patient in first class," he said anxiously. "Could you take a look at him?"

The man was fortyish, rotund and balding and dressed in a Khaki bush jacket. He was a wealthy Californian who had been big-game hunting in Kenya.

"Are you taking antimalarials?" I asked him.

"No," he said. "My white hunter told me there was no malaria in the areas we were hunting in."

"Where were you?"

"Down on the Tana River."

"I know the area," I said. "I first saw it ten years ago. There is a lot of malaria there."

The white hunter was absolutely wrong. But the bad advice he gave is not unusual because people living in malarial areas consider the disease in relative terms and not absolute ones. They often think of the dry season as being malaria-free, which it isn't. The disease is less frequent then because there are fewer mosquitoes around to transmit it, but it is still present. And they think of the rainy season as the time for malaria because the increased mosquito populations transmit the disease more readily. "Whether it's the dry or rainy season, you've got to take antimalarials," I told the passenger as I examined him. My exam didn't turn anything up except that he had a fever of 103. I was certain he had malaria. But I couldn't prove it without a blood smear.

"I can treat you with chloroquine, which I have in my bag," I told him, "but I think you should get off here in Dakar and rest for a day or so before traveling back to the States."

"Can't do that. I've got to be in Los Angeles to close a deal this afternoon."

"The airline will take care of you," I assured him. "And I'll give you the names of two doctors I know here who are very competent. You may not need them, but just in case."

I gave the passenger a loading dose of four chloroquine tablets and told him to take two more in six hours and then two in twenty-four and two in forty-eight hours. "But I think you should rest here," I said. I went up to the cockpit to speak with the crew. The pilot had the handbook of regulations spread out on his lap.

"He ought to get off here and rest for a day or so," I said.

"But he refuses," the pilot answered. "And I don't want to take the chance of going out over the Atlantic with someone who might get very sick on the way. We fly up to the Azores and after that it's four hours to the nearest landing field if we have to make an emergency landing."

"I don't think he should travel," I said, "not because something might happen to him, but because someone with malaria should rest in bed for a day or so."

The pilot picked up on that. "You think he can travel then without any risk. If that's the case we can fly out with him if you sign a waiver certifying he's healthy enough to travel."

"You're twisting my words," I said. "I can't guarantee nothing will happen to him en route. Chances are he'll be all right. But I'm

218

not a crystal-ball gazer. The conventional medical wisdom is he should stay put in bed for a couple of days."

The passenger refused to listen to reason and during the hour which elapsed since I gave him the chloroquine began feeling better. The crew was afraid of forcing him to get off because he was a VIP. The local manager even offered to put him up in his home. But the passenger was adamant. "I have to be in Los Angeles in the afternoon," he kept saying.

Finally the manager decided to call in a local French doctor. Another hour went by while we waited for him to arrive. I stepped out of the plane and walked out onto the tarmac where the ground crew asked me in French what was going on. "Un cas du paludisme," I said. "Comment!" one of them exclaimed. "Ce n'est pas grand chose ça." His reaction didn't surprise me because, from an African's perspective, malaria is a common everyday disease.

The French doctor finally arrived with the manager and came shuffling out to the plane in slippers. We knew each other.

"Imperato!" he said. "What are you up to now?"

"Malaria." I laughed back.

"Ah, that's no problem. I'll blast him with a shot of quinine."

"I've already given him chloroquine," I said as we climbed up the stairs to the plane. "You'll make him toxic."

"Ah, so what? A little toxicity will make him remember it better. You Americans are always talking about drug toxicity. That's all I read about in your journals. You ought to be like us French. Live a little adventurously."

He gave the passenger a shot in the buttocks in full view of the other passengers, with the reading light beamed in on one cheek. "Maybe you shouldn't expose him like that," I said in French. "Why not?" said my colleague, wiping the tip of his needle off with a piece of cotton. I cringed and thought about its questionable sterility. "They all have asses like his. Maybe not as big, but not much different." And on that note he gave the injection. Then he signed the waiver and before going out onto the stairway platform said, "When you come back, let's have dinner. You can fill me in on what happens to the big-game hunter."

Nice of him, I thought. If this patient develops problems en route, it will be my problem.

219

Fortunately, the passenger recovered midway across the Atlantic. But he complained of severe ringing in his ears. It is one of the side reactions to heavy doses of quinine and chloroquine. "It's the price you have to pay," I told him, "for not taking antimalarials and for wanting to be in Los Angeles this afternoon."

CHAPTER 18

SEARCHING FOR THE FLU

As the days grew colder, the staff talked about nothing but the flu. It didn't surprise me. But I had been damned surprised eleven months earlier, at the tail end of the winter season, when I found everyone so preoccupied with the flu. "Why is everyone so uptight about the flu?" I asked Dr. Chaves at the time. A big to-do about nothing, I thought.

"After all," I told him smugly, "in Africa influenza epidemics came and went and nobody paid any attention to them."

"Maybe that's how it is in Africa," he replied, "but here, the flu is an important disease to everyone,"

In time I came to realize that Chaves was right. But during those early days, just back from Africa, my perspective on epidemics was strongly conditioned by having dealt with diseases which killed most who got them. I found it hard to get all worked up over a disease like the flu. Of course I came to understand the flu is a fickle disease. Some years it causes epidemics, other years it hardly makes itself known. Some strains of the flu virus cause significant mortality, other do not. The Center for Disease Control in Atlanta estimates that flu epidemics occurring between 1968 and 1978 were responsible for 150,000 deaths. Most remember or at least have heard of the flu epidemic of 1918. It was called the Spanish influenza in the United States in the mistaken belief that it started in Spain. But in Spain it was called the French influenza and in Japan the American influenza. We know that this disease was in the United States before it ever got to Spain, so the names reveal more about national feelings and mistaken perceptions than they do about the origins of the disease. The world's population was approximately two billion in 1918 and it's estimated that half came down with this flu. And of that number twenty-two million are thought to have died. Although flu epidemics have occurred at regular intervals since 1918, none has equaled that holocaust. Most epidemics make a lot of people sick and miserable. But they do not carry high fatality rates compared to diseases like cholera and epidemic meningitis.

But flu epidemics do have a number of effects other than medical ones on a complex technological society like ours. "Just think of the impact of a wide-scale epidemic," Chaves said, "on critical service-providing organizations and institutions. Employees out with the flu translate into high absenteeism rates which have serious repercussions in places like hospitals, in fire and police departments and in the service areas. Think for a moment what happens when half the employees of a hospital are home sick with the flu."

I had to admit to him that it sounded sobering. It was just that in Africa flu was considered a minor nuisance. And as far as its impact there on vital services was concerned, well, we never gave it a thought. We didn't have many services to "cripple." Demands for services were low and people didn't complain even when they were stopped altogether.

The influenza virus has adapted itself to man extremely well. It infects the cells of the respiratory tract where it grows and multiplies. Usually it doesn't cause any more harm than to create a sore throat, runny nose, cough and perhaps laryngitis. Those affected by it in this mild way feel achy, have a fever for a few days and quickly go through boxes of tissues. Occasionally, the flu virus can cause pneumonia or predispose the victim to pneumonia-causing bacteria. And often it causes an illness so mild the person doesn't realize he's had the flu.

The flu virus is spread from one person to another by coughing, sneezing or just breathing. But as it passes from one person to another and through the population, man's cells build up antibodies

222

to it. These defense substances can quickly destroy the virus. This means that if the virus stays around in a community long enough, most people will develop these antibodies and eventually the virus will be killed off. Epidemiologists have known for a number of years, as have other scientists, that the influenza virus deals with this enormous obstacle to its own survival in an efficient manner. The virus present in the noses and throats of victims at any given time is not identical in terms of genetic makeup. A single infection is caused by billions of virus particles. Most of these are identical, but a few aren't. These slightly different virus particles are called mutants. Mutants can't be detected because they are a minority in the influenza virus population. They begin to take over, however, as antibodies build up and start destroying the dominant virus particles. These mutants are not totally immune to the antibodies that efficiently kill their fellows, but they can withstand an attack and survive. This lifesaving mechanism on the part of the flu virus is called "antigenic drift." Mutants tend to emerge every two to three years. When they do, people who have already had the flu may get it again. But since the mutants are so similar to their now disappeared dominant relatives, they are also affected by the person's existing antibodies. The resulting bout of flu is usually not so severe. Recent examples of mutants include the London flu, the Port Chalmers flu, the A Victoria flu and the Russian flu.

Every ten years or so, worldwide flu epidemics occur. They are caused by flu viruses which are not affected by all of the antibodies built up by antigenic drift. This means that, unlike the mutants, they are not cousins but unrelated to the flu viruses which have been around before. It is not fully understood how these new flu viruses develop and where they come from. But many scientists suspect that they develop in swine. It has long been known that swine are infected by human flu viruses. Scientists theorize that when a virus is driven out of circulation in the human population by antibodies, it seeks a safe haven in swine. In time the mutants which have replaced it in humans will join it, being driven out of humans by antibodies. Some speculate that all of these first cousins combine together and pool their genetic material to create a totally new and different virus which is unaffected by any of the antibodies circulating in the human population. Once ready, this new virus comes out of swine and infects humans, causing a worldwide epi-

223

demic. This device of the flu virus is called "antigenic shift." It occurs about every decade. It is a different mechanism from "antigenic drift." Examples of it in recent times are the Asian flu of 1957 and the Hong Kong flu of 1968.

The reason why many scientists became alarmed in February 1976 with the appearance of the swine-flu virus at Fort Dix, New Jersey, was because it surfaced at a time when the ten-year period of the Hong Kong flu was just about up. They assumed that it was the virus that was going to cause the next worldwide epidemic. In retrospect, their guess was wrong. But at the time, their guess was as good as any. The swine-flu virus is totally different from its immediate predecessors and is also a relative of the virus which caused the terrible epidemic of 1918. But aside from the Fort Dix episode, it didn't cause any epidemics. Scientists have since learned that there is not one swine-flu virus but several which are closely related to one another and that they are around all the time, causing mild sporadic cases of the flu, especially in people exposed to swine. This recent experience illustrates how difficult it is to predict which virus is going to take over at the end of a given ten-year period. It also shows that we still have a lot to learn about flu viruses and their behavior.

The World Health Organization has set up eighty-five influenza-virus reference laboratories in fifty-five countries in an attempt to keep track of the new strains which appear all the time. A World Influenza Center has also been set up to coordinate the efforts of all these laboratories. The center screens hundreds of specimens each year sent to it from all over the world. Tests are conducted to determine if the specimens contain mutants, currently known strains or completely new and as yet unknown viruses. Obviously, the reason for all this screening is to save lives. To do this, vaccines must contain killed virus particles identical to those which are currently causing the flu. Vaccines made from previously dominant strains do offer some protection against the mutants which emerge every two to three years, but the protection is not very high. Hence mutants must be uncovered as quickly as possible, their epidemiologic activity in the population studied and assessed and a decision made about incorporating them into the yearly vaccine.

The New York City Health Department's Bureau of Infectious

Disease Control is one of the most crucial flu-monitoring stations in the country. New York City is an international transportation hub. Over ten thousand passengers come into Kennedy International Airport every day, not to mention the thousands who arrive at other airports and by train and road. A mutant flu virus or a completely new strain turns up quickly in a place where crowds are dense and human contacts frequent and close. So now it was my job to monitor the flu and to lead the search for mutants and new viruses.

The flu season usually runs from November through February and peaks in late December and early January. Each year, all across the country, mobile teams of vaccinators go into senior-citizen centers and nursing homes. And vaccinations are given by private physicians, clinics, hospitals and health centers so that the elderly and the chronically ill can be protected from the flu. To be effective, the vaccines have to be given before the flu season starts. That was why we had sent out the vaccinators of the bureau's Immunization Program in September and October. We also distributed free vaccine to physicians and other health providers.

But this year, 1972, things were different: a new mutant was expected. The old one had been around for about three and a half years and the majority of people in the country had antibodies to it. A mutant, known popularly as the London flu, had appeared in England in early 1972. It spread far and wide in Europe and now we were on watch, waiting to see if it would spread to the United States and in so doing become the dominant strain. There was no way of knowing whether this would happen or not, just as there was no sure way of knowing in 1976 what the swine-flu virus was going to do. For that reason, the London-flu virus hadn't been incorporated into the vaccine we were then using. But that vaccine did contain some first cousins to the London-flu virus, thus providing a certain degree of protection in the event it struck.

Bill Herbert had been through one flu season already and knew the ropes as a flu detective. I may have been his teacher most of the year, but now our roles were reversed. "The newspapers, radio and television stations take an intense interest in the flu," he warned me. "You've got to be on your toes all the time with them." Flu stories make good copy because everyone can be affected by the disease. Reporters tended toward hyperbole when it came to the flu and if I weren't careful, Bill said, "they'll be yelling there's an epidemic even if it's just one case we've told them about."

Individual cases of the flu aren't reported and tabulated nationally by the Center for Disease Control. "Wouldn't it make things a lot easier for a flu detective if they were?" many often ask. It wouldn't. Most flu cases are diagnosed by patients themselves and by their physicians who may or may not physically see them. More often than not the doctor will handle the problem over the phone by saying, "Sounds like the flu. Stay in bed, drink plenty of fluids; take aspirin every four hours and if you're not better in two or three days call me." While the margin of error in making the diagnosis isn't great, it's large enough to reduce the value of reporting cases to local health departments and to the Center for Disease Control. Many virus diseases mimic the flu in the symptoms they cause. People who think they have the flu may not. If their cases were reported to local health departments it would result in what epidemiologists call "false positive reports," or reports of something that isn't really there.

How then does an epidemiologist keep track of the flu? I didn't have the foggiest idea! But as Director of the Bureau, I learned fast. And I was in a good place to learn because New York City and a few other states were the only places at the time which had complex influenza surveillance systems. That year when I was a novice myself, the Center for Disease Control began setting up a national flu-detection program, incorporating the activities which until that time had been going on in New York City and a few other places like California. In a sense, then, I had many classmates among my fellow epidemiologists throughout the country.

The National Influenza Surveillance System functions throughout the year, but intensifies its activities between November and February—the "influenza season." Health departments all across the United States send detailed information to the system on forms which make it regular and uniform. This information along with statistical data are then sent back to health departments and public-health officials in published form in the *Morbidity and Mortality Weekly Report*, known to insiders by the acronym *MMWR*. This publication is a sort of professional newsletter produced by the Center for Disease Control primarily for the benefit of the nation's medical detectives and other public-health experts. But it is also sent to doctors, nurses and other people working in the broad field of medicine who have an interest in communicable diseases.

Medical detectives have long observed that one of the first things that happens when the flu arrives on the scene is a sharp rise in the number of people going to emergency rooms and outpatient depart- ments of hospitals, especially in large cities where many people use these instead of private physicians.

This part of the influenza-tracking system, *hospital surveillance*, had been put into place in New York City several years before by one of my predecessors. Pointing to the red pins which showed their location on a large wall map of New York City, Bill said, "I'll personally call the three largest every day and the clerks will call the rest. That way we'll know what's going on from day to day. If we see a sudden and dramatic rise in the numbers of people going to emergency rooms," Bill said, "then chances are there's a new flu strain around." This may be strong circumstantial evidence, but it isn't absolute proof. But Bill explained that the game plan was then to go to an emergency room with a sudden increase in visits and try to isolate the virus from people coming in with flu symp- toms.

The second part of the surveillance system is *industrial absentee- ism.* "Last year Chaves and I set up a program with twelve large corporations in the city. They all have medical departments and together monitor about 120,000 employees."

"Smart," I said. "When the flu hits, people stay home and the medical departments register a sudden increase in absenteeism."

"Right, but," Bill added, "the catch is that toward Christmas when the flu often peaks, people stay out to do Christmas shop- ping. So it's not too useful an indicator. But it's worth trying."

The third activity, *school absenteeism*, also had a chink in its ar- mor. Infection rates for the flu tend to be highest among primary- and secondary-school children. This is because children, unlike adults, usually don't have any carryover immunity from previous flu infections. But changes in truancy rates may be affecting re- sults.

"The only clear and certain measure of influenza activity is the one we get too late to be of much immediate help, *pneumonia mor- tality*," Bill explained.

227

Pneumonia is a frequent complication of influenza and causes death about two weeks after the original influenza illness. Death certificates are filed with the New York City Health Department and the number of deaths due to pneumonia tabulated on a weekly basis.

"Here's the chart the statisticians make up," Bill said, holding up a large piece of cardboard. A broad gray band starting like the crest of a hill in January descended into a trough in the spring and summer months and then began climbing again in the fall. "This gray band is the expected deaths due to pneumonia," Bill said, continuing his lecture. "The red line is the actual number of deaths. As you can see, it hasn't gone above the gray curve. If it does then we know something's happening."

"Pretty straightforward," I said. "If the actual number of deaths goes above the tolerance zone we've got an influenza epidemic."

"Right."

Going over to his desk, Bill pulled out another pile of graphs. "These are the graphs showing antibody levels to the different strains of virus."

"How do we get them?"

"Easy. The labs run antibody tests on the serum collected from people getting blood tests for syphilis down at the marriage bureau. Everybody getting married in this town has got to get a test for syphilis. Our guys take those samples and pool them together and then run antibody levels on the pool once a week."

"That's an ingenious idea."

"Pretty nifty. We're the only place in the country that does it." Pointing to the latest graph he said, "You see, about 60 percent of the people have good antibodies to the Hong Kong virus of 1968."

"That's damn high."

"Sure is. No chance we're going to have any trouble with this virus again. If the London flu is a first cousin, then we're home safe. These antibodies will knock the steam out of it. But if it's a second or third cousin, well then, who knows? We could have a big one."

"How about isolating the virus?"

"Harder than hell. It's only been done once before."

"But that's the hard proof we really need, isn't it?"

"Sure it is, but it's not easy to come by."

228

"Maybe we'll be lucky this year."

There it was, an elaborate detection system for the flu. It impressed me as being a network composed of a lot of indirect but very useful measurements—"indicators" as they're known in jargon to medical detectives. Of course, whenever reporters ask, "How many cases of the flu have occurred in the city this year so far?" we still can't give them a firm answer. But we can tell them a lot of other things about the flu. And most importantly, this information enables us to prepare the right kind of vaccine for the following year. The vaccines come out a year after the new strain has had a first swipe at the population. Too late to be of help to those who get the flu the first year, but useful for the next two or three years when the new strain reigns supreme.

In late November I received a call from the chief physician of the Riker's Island Prison Infirmary. "I need some advice about a patient with hepatitis," he said. After I gave him what he wanted, I asked, "Have you seen any flu cases among the prisoners?"

"I've seen a lot of colds, but we always get this sort of thing out here this time of year."

"What kind of symptoms do they have?"

He grew impatient. "Haven't you ever had a cold?"

"Okay, how many people have you seen with colds?"

"Oh, I'd say about a couple of hundred. Some with fevers. Must be some kind of cold virus."

Zebras flashed. I couldn't take this information at face value.

"Do you mind if we come out to Riker's Island and look at the prisoners?"

"Come on out if you want to waste your time."

Bill and I were out at the prison by noon. We found fourteen prisoners in the infirmary who had fevers, body aches and headaches.

"This sure looks like the flu," I said to Bill.

"I'll say. Cold viruses don't cause this kind of disease."

The chief physician didn't agree with us, but he let us take some specimens from the prisoner-patients. Bill and I had them gargle a sterile solution and spit it out into sterile containers and then we rinsed their nasal passages with the same sterile solution. This gave us mucus from the respiratory passages, and if the flu virus was there it could be recovered in the laboratory. We got ten specimens in all and took them to the laboratories. "It will take about ten days to isolate the virus," the director of the virology laboratory told us, "*if* the virus is there."

Over the next week all of the statistical indices stayed in the normal range. There was nothing to suggest that there was any significant flu activity going on in the city.

But on December 8, the director of virology called me from the labs and said, "It's influenza all right. But I can't tell you if it's the London flu or not. I have to send the virus isolate to CDC because they have the identifying antisera."

"We can't say anything yet," Bill said, when I told him about the lab results. "I'm almost sure it's the London flu. We're going to see those statistics skyrocket in about two weeks or so."

Another week went by and than late one afternoon I got a call from the virus laboratory of the CDC. "The viruses you isolated are A/England/42/72," he said, giving me the technical name for the London-flu virus.

"Wow, that's some coup," Bill said, almost jumping into the air. "What a stroke of luck. We found it. It's here."

The fact that it was here became evident within the next couple of days. Several hundred prisoners were brought into the infirmary and absenteeism rates in schools and businesses began climbing. At the same time the number of visits to emergency rooms and outpatient departments swung upward. But from what we could gather at this early stage, the London flu was more like a first cousin to its predecessor than a distant relative. The epidemic didn't have the makings of a major disaster because so many people's antibodies from the 1968 Hong Kong flu were giving them protection against the London flu. The press was informed and in spite of what I had been prepared to expect handled the epidemic calmly. *"City Has Eye On A New Flu Called London"* was one of the early headlines in a New York newspaper. That summed it up. As the month of January moved on, the rates climbed, but not to staggering heights. The red line on the pneumonia mortality chart ran only ten deaths above the expected range. "No big deal," Bill said one day after looking over all of the statistical evidence. "On the Herbert-Imperato Scale, this is a mild one" he said laughingly one day. "I'd rate it three points out of ten."

We forwarded our findings to the Center for Disease Control in

Atlanta and they disseminated it throughout the country. Pretty soon the London flu popped up all over the country. But everywhere it was the same story. This first cousin to the Hong Kong flu of 1968 wasn't causing much trouble.

But what was clear was that the London flu virus had now replaced the Hong Kong virus. This meant that the flu vaccine for the following flu season, 1973–74, had to contain the London-flu virus in place of its predecessor, the Hong Kong virus. And so in early 1973, the pharmaceutical houses began producing this new vaccine so it would be ready for the upcoming season. By late August this vaccine, which took about six months to make, was ready for distribution and administration to the elderly and other high-risk patients. Like all flu vaccines it provided protection for only about six months. So it had to be administered in September and October to take advantage of this period of protection.

But we were outfoxed again by the flu! No sooner was the vaccine being administered than a new strain appeared, called the Port Chalmers flu. It was only distantly related to the London flu and the Hong Kong flu, so the vaccine didn't provide much protection against it, nor did antibodies developed from previous infections with either virus. It swept through places like New York City with fury. In place of the ten excess deaths from pneumonia a week which we had seen during the London flu, almost a hundred excess deaths per week occurred. The epidemic was massive and lethal. By January 1974 the Port Chalmers flu had taken over the stage and the London flu disappeared.

Armed with this information, gathered by epidemiologists all over the country, the pharmaceutical houses replaced the London-flu virus in the vaccine with the Port Chalmers virus. When the 1974–75 flu season rolled around, the Port Chalmers virus stayed on the scene and no new virus appeared. So the vaccine protected those who received it. But no sooner was the 1975 flu season over, around February, than a new mutant appeared. Called A/Victoria, it was named like all flu viruses after the place where it was first isolated. By the end of 1975, when the flu season came around again, A/Victoria had the upper hand and was pushing Port Chalmers off the scene.

It is unusual for so many mutants to appear in such quick succession. Usually a mutant rules supreme for a few years. And that is what happened once A/Victoria appeared. It remained the dominant virus until 1978 when the Russian flu moved across the world into the United States.

"It's a crazy business," Bill said. "And the general public wonders why we don't have a better handle on it. Why these viruses are coming along faster than a convoy of commuter trains!"

Several years later Bill called me from California where he had returned to complete his training. At the time I was the First Deputy Health Commissioner and Chairman of the New York City Swine Influenza Immunization Task Force. It was the fall of 1976, at the height of the swine-flu controversy. "Boy, it's a far cry from the old days of London flu," he said. "It was hard enough then trying to predict what was going to happen."

Flu was the top story of the year. My office practically became a radio and television studio. Every day witnessed a procession of radio and television interviewers and journalists from the press.

If I hadn't known anything about public relations before, I was certainly learning now. I found that the key was to try to explain complex technical and medical knowledge in laymen's terms. It had to be concise, understandable and preferably black or white. This wasn't easy to do since each passing day ushered in a new crisis. As the director of the largest single swine-flu immunization program in the country, I had to calm people's anxieties and concerns and at the same time explain my own position that the immunization was being made available to them but that I wasn't overly enthusiastic about it. The decision to be immunized had to be their own.

National experts had made a decision early in 1976 to immunize the entire population against swine flu. This seemed reasonable to me. But as the summer months appeared and no cases of swine flu surfaced in the southern hemisphere, which was then experiencing its winter season, I and many other epidemiologists had doubts that the disease would become an epidemic threat. I favored a change in policy to recommending that the elderly and chronically ill be immunized, not the entire population. However, the national policy formulated by the Center for Disease Control early in the year remained unaltered. Public credibility in that policy, which recommended immunizing everyone, clearly waned at this point. I conducted a number of interview surveys throughout the city at this time and discovered that only 16.1 percent of those questioned had received an inoculation against swine flu. Those who hadn't and didn't intend to amounted to 53.4 percent and those who were afraid to 33.5 percent. Some 12.8 percent had been advised not to get it by their family doctor and 2.2 percent had no reason. This survey was conducted in mid-November, 1976, a time when only 5 percent of New York City's population had been immunized against the swine flu. It clearly told me that people weren't going to be immunized. And by the time the program ended in December, only 639,144 people in the city had received shots out of a population of close to eight million.

The policy of the New York City Department of Health was that it would make immunizations available in scores of clinics and from mobile clinics and distribute vaccine to hospitals and doctors, but that the individual had to make his or her own decision about being immunized. The reason for this policy was simply in response to the facts as they emerged over the months prior to the beginning of the immunization program in October 1976. And those facts said loud and clear that swine flu was always around, causing a case here and a case there, but that it was mild and unlikely to cause an epidemic.

Searching for the flu is like looking into a hazy crystal ball. And this is really amazing, in a century marked by tremendous medical progress. Here's flu, one of the oldest diseases, affecting most people at some time in their lives, and we have only imprecise tools for tracking it, educated guesses for predicting its future behavior, mediocre vaccines for protecting people against it and absolutely no way of curing it. Dr. William Foege, the director of the Center for Disease Control, summed it up when he said that the flu is a very humbling disease because the expected doesn't often happen and the unexpected does.

CHAPTER 19

EASTER DINNER

Soon after the London Flu disappeared from New York in early 1973, I got back to planning the reorganization of the bureau. I held several meetings with Eleanor Lambertsen, dean of the Cornell University–New York Hospital School of Nursing and Dr. George Reader, chairman of the Department of Public Health at Cornell University Medical College. They had already trained a number of our public-health nurses to be pediatric nurse associates. During a year of training, the nurses were given intensive exposure to the diagnosis and treatment of the problems of children. And equipped with these new skills they worked in schools and the Health Department's child health stations.

Since nurses had performed so well as substitute pediatricians there was no reason they couldn't be trained as epidemiologists. The Cornell staff and the Commissioner of Health shared my enthusiasm. Eventually union opposition and staff suspicions dwindled too. I felt that things were beginning to take shape. Over the next couple of months I held frequent meetings with Miss Margaret O'Brien, the director of the Bureau of Public Health Nursing and drew up standards for selecting the nurse candidates for the program. We decided that they should all have a bachelor's degree in nursing and have maintained at least a B average during their formal training. In addition we were going to require that they all have at least ten years of public-health nursing experience. And since the nurses were to be selected from within the Department of Health, this meant that they would all know the ropes inside and out. But in spite of all of this progress, there were months of planning and patient waiting ahead.

At the time I was busy making all these plans, a sixty-year-old woman was also busy preparing a large Easter Sunday dinner for her family in Brooklyn. Maria Mazzio always made lasagna for Easter and her sauce was her own from beginning to end. She grew her own tomatoes during the summer months and then canned them at home when they were ripe. She stored the large tins of tomatoes in a cool corner of the basement. Maria had been canning tomatoes for years, in fact ever since she was a little girl. She had learned to do it from her mother and grandmother. Everyone raved about the quality of her sauce. There was nothing like it. And when she served her lasagna this Easter, as usual everyone complimented her and told her how wonderful the sauce was.

On Monday night, Maria, who everyone said was as strong as a horse, felt dizzy and weak. "I think I have the flu," she told her eldest daughter Teresa over the phone.

"You'd better go to bed," Teresa advised her, "I'll call you in the morning to see how you are."

When Teresa called her mother in the morning she found she wasn't any better. In fact she was a lot worse. She sounded hoarse and told Teresa, "My eyes are blurred and I can't keep my eyelids open."

Teresa didn't think this sounded like the flu so she rushed over to her mother's house. "I don't like the way you're breathing, Ma. I think I'd better call Dr. Williams."

"Bring her over," Dr. Williams said over the phone. "I can't say what it is from what you tell me."

By the time Teresa got her mother to the doctor's office, things were worse. "She may have heart failure," Dr. Williams whispered to Teresa after he had completed his examination. "I'm going to hospitalize her for some tests."

Bergen Hospital was a small proprietary hospital which has long since been closed. It was a pretty, little building put up in the late 1950s by a group of local general practitioners. But like so many institutions of its kind it was cut off from the mainstream of medicine and its aging staff grew less competent with each passing year. Maria was put into a comfortable private room which had a view of nearby Prospect Park, now ablaze with cherry blossoms, soft fresh grass and budding trees. The nurses were courteous and Dr. Williams came to see Maria twice the first day she was hospitalized. Blood and urine samples were taken for tests and x-rays made of Maria's lungs. When the results came back the next day, they were all normal, but Maria was worse. She had completely lost her voice and couldn't swallow.

Dr. Williams called in a friend of his who was on the staff of the hospital. "I don't know what to make of it," he told his colleague. "The electrocardiogram is normal, chest x-ray normal and all the blood and urine tests normal. But she's in respiratory distress and has lost her voice and can't open her eyes."

Dr. Williams's colleague went in and examined Maria and then reviewed her chart. "It must be some kind of virus," he said. "I don't know what else could do this. Why don't you give her some oxygen and see how she does in the next few days."

"Good idea," Williams said, still unsure about what Maria really had. He had thought of getting a specialist in from one of the larger nearby teaching hospitals, but Bergen Hospital didn't have any formal arrangement with those institutions. And he himself didn't know anyone professionally except those who were on the staff of Bergen.

The oxygen didn't do Maria much good. "I'm afraid it looks hopeless," he confessed to Teresa a few hours later. "She has a rare form of heart failure which doesn't respond to oxygen or to the digitalis heart medicine I've given her."

"How could that be?" Teresa queried. "She's never been sick a day in her life. And you said the electrocardiogram was normal. How could she have heart failure with a normal electrocardiogram?"

"Sometimes a heart attack in the back of the heart isn't picked up on the electrocardiogram," he explained to Teresa. And she believed him.

Maria Mazzio died peacefully in an oxygen tent a few hours later. "She didn't suffer too much," Dr. Williams said, trying to comfort Teresa and the other members of the family. He went down to

237

the admitting office to make out the death certificate. The clerk had already filled out most of the form except for the confidential part of it listing the cause and contributing causes of death. Dr. Williams felt some flashes of doubt as he started filling in the form.

Maria's remains were taken to a local funeral parlor where they were laid out for a three-day wake. Toward the evening of the first night of the wake, Teresa became hoarse and had trouble keeping her eyelids open. "I'm getting the same thing Mama had," she said to her husband.

"Don't be silly," he replied. "You're just upset. After all, it's been a terrible ordeal for you."

Teresa was concerned enough to call Dr. Williams's answering service and left a message for him to call her back as soon as possible. When he did an hour later, she told him her vision was blurred, her voice hoarse and her eyelids droopy. "Now take it easy," he said. "You've been under a lot of stress," he went on to comfort her. "Let me speak with your husband," he said when he had finished speaking with her.

"I think she's having an hysterical reaction," he told him.

"That's what I thought, Doc."

"It's very common. People think they're getting the same thing as the person who has just died. Heart failure isn't contagious. You understand."

"I'll call in a prescription for a tranquilizer to whatever pharmacy is near there."

"Sure enough, there's one on Atlantic and Court streets. It's called the Long Island."

Dr. Williams called the pharmacy and Teresa took the tranquilizers as prescribed. But she didn't improve. Her symptoms weren't as bad as her mother's but they were unmistakably there. Some of the relatives thought she was faking it, others that she was just hysterical. She managed to go through the second day of the wake and the final day of the funeral.

But after coming home from the cemetery, Teresa felt too weak to participate in the dinner which the other members of the family arranged. Teresa wasn't known to be a person who complained so her husband began wondering about Dr. Williams's diagnosis. He decided to take her to the emergency room of a hospital near their home in the southern part of Brooklyn. The intern who examined her was a foreigner and Teresa's husband had a hard time understanding what he said. But he did pick up that Teresa had a viral infection and that a few days of bed rest would cure it.

Teresa's husband wasn't satisfied with that. He took her to the emergency room of Newkirk Hospital, a large municipal hospital which serves part of the borough of Brooklyn. She was seen by a young intern, Dr. Donald Levine. He had never seen an illness like this one. He didn't know what to make of it. But he suspected it was something contagious since Teresa's husband told him all about Maria Mazzio's illness. Levine, like other interns in the city, knew he could consult with the Bureau of Infectious Disease Control and so he put a call through to me.

After he told me the story, I said, "Both she and her mother presented with paralysis of the cranial nerves."

"That's right," he said, "It's really weird."

"It may be weird," I said, "but it's typical of one disease. Botulism!"

"Gee, I thought of botulism. But then I said to myself it can't be. Who ever sees botulism anymore?"

"Your hunch was right," I said. "Always follow your instincts. Otherwise you're going to miss the zebras that come along. Now look, we've got to get some big doses of antitoxin into her right away if we're going to save her. I'll have a messenger bring it over to you from the department's laboratories. And at this end we've got to find out where they got it from because others might have eaten the toxin."

Botulism is a severe intoxication which people get whenever they ingest foods which are contaminated with the toxin of a bacterium known as *Clostridium botulinum*. The botulinum toxins are among the most powerful poisons known. The bacterium grows and produces toxin in foods which have been inadequately processed and heated. *Clostridium botulinum* is what is known as an anaerobic organism, meaning that it thrives in the absence of oxygen. Canned and bottled foods are generally anaerobic because all of the air is taken out of the containers during the sealing process. There are six strains of the organism, lettered A through F, and the toxins they produce attack the body's cranial nerves which control vital functions such as swallowing, speech, sight and breathing. Maria Mazzio didn't die from heart failure but from paralysis of the diaphragm, the giant muscle which separates the chest from the abdomen and which enables us to breathe.

Most cases of botulism in the United States result from the ingestion of toxin-contaminated home-canned vegetables, fruits and fish. *Clostridium botulinum* is a microbe which is found in many places in nature. Type E, for example, is often found in the intestinal tract of fishes, in lake-shore mud and in sea-bottom silt. Even though home canners follow instructions carefully, their foods can always be contaminated by the organism. Once inside an airless sealed can or jar, the microbe thrives and produces its toxin which can survive for a very long period of time and resist refrigeration. Some strains of botulinum produce enzymes which alter the taste of the food. But others do not, meaning that the food tastes, smells and looks perfectly fine.

In recent years, a number of commercially canned products have been contaminated with botulinum toxins which have resulted in widespread epidemics. The most famous of these were due to contaminated tuna fish, mushroom soup and vichyssoise soup.

I had no way of knowing the source of this intoxication, nor how many people had been exposed to it. If it were from a commercially prepared product the ramifications were very severe, since thousands of people would be at risk. I notified the Center for Disease Control and they told me that there hadn't been any cases reported in the rest of the country. This didn't rule out a commercial source, but it did point the finger toward a home-canned product. I went to the Mazzio home and interviewed Teresa's husband and Maria's widower. They told me about Maria's home-canned tomatoes.

"But if it's the canned tomatoes, then why didn't the rest of us get sick?" Teresa's husband asked.

"The toxin is killed by ten minutes of boiling. Chances are that all of you ate the sauce after the toxin had been destroyed.

"That's it," he replied. "Tessie and Mama cooked the sauce on Easter and they kept tasting it all the time. I'll bet they ate it before it boiled. Sure, they must have. They always tasted it right after opening the can."

Although the tomatoes were suspect number one, I had to prove it. I took samples from the Mazzio home and sent sanitary inspectors to bring in the score of cans down in the basement. Eventually we found botulinum toxin in several of them.

Maria, her mother and grandmother had been home canning for close to a century. Nothing like this had ever happened.

"Why now?" Teresa's husband asked. "How come nothing happened before?"

"They were just lucky," I said. "The organism happened to be around this time and got into the cans. They weren't heated enough to kill it off."

I gave all the members of the Mazzio family antitoxin as a precautionary measure and none of them came down with botulism. But at Newkirk Hospital, Teresa's condition grew worse in spite of the large doses of antitoxin which Dr. Levine gave her. "The toxin's had several days' start on us," he said dejectedly over the phone. "If only she had come in a few days earlier. It would have been a snap to save her."

Teresa died in spite of all the efforts Dr. Levine made to save her. Defective home canning and the tasting of contaminated uncooked tomatoes were the two fatal variables which led to the intoxication of Teresa and her mother. Botulism is a very rare disease in the United States and only a handful of cases occur each year. It's about as rare a zebra as one can find and understandably most doctors have never seen a case. The diagnosis isn't easy to make for those who aren't familiar with the disease. And even if the diagnosis is made early and the patient promptly treated with antitoxin, there is no guarantee that he'll recover. So the possibility exists that Teresa and her mother might have died even if they had been treated early. No one can say for sure.

CHAPTER 20

FULL-FLEDGED EPIDEMIOLOGIST

By the summer of 1973, I had been directing the bureau for a year and a half. During that time I mastered an enormous body of hard scientific facts about the communicable diseases, building upon my African knowledge. But knowledge wasn't enough; it certainly wasn't the element which gave me the sense that I had finally arrived, that I was a full-fledged epidemiologist. What really gave me that sense more than anything else was a strong inner feeling of self-confidence, which built up gradually with each new, difficult, and sometimes horrifying experience. And now I felt secure with my reasoning and comfortable with my decisions. It wasn't that doubts never crossed my mind. There was always doubt. But knowledge and self-confidence are a great combination and enabled me to function even when doubt too was present.

Similar problems arose time and again—a case of hepatitis in a school, food poisoning at a church picnic, measles in a day-care center, an isolated case of polio, staphylococcal infections in nurseries and a host of what we called garden-variety outbreaks. I felt few hesitations now about what to do, what to look for, and surprised even myself sometimes with my ability to guess accurately in advance the probable sources of infections and how they spread. Microbes have standard characteristics and the epidemics they cause have predictable patterns of behavior. Being the chief epidemiologist of New York City gave me a season ticket to the most active communicable-disease theater in the world. I got to know each microbe's repertoire by heart once I had seen a variety perform in a broad selection of plays.

At about this time in fact, a problem arose in which my self-confidence and knowledge proved their strength in the face of opposition.

A resident physician called me from a large medical center and said, "We've just admitted a woman with severe pneumonia. It looks like viral pneumonia."

I knew from those few words that the woman didn't have an ordinary viral pneumonia. This medical center is one of the best in the country and the resident wouldn't call unless they were stumped. Had the call come from a smaller, lesser-quality hospital, my thoughts would have gone in a different direction.

"You don't think it's an ordinary viral pneumonia?"

"Er, well, not really. You see, her three-year-old son died this morning here from the same type of pneumonia. We were sort of wondering if there's anything like this going on in the city."

This was his way of saying they didn't know what it was. Physicians at the large teaching medical centers rarely would admit to me and Bill Herbert that they needed help. Those calling from the smaller hospitals would blurt out, "I don't know what it is. I need help." But such candor rarely came out of the ivory towers. Their calls were more cautious probes, attempts to pick our brains for what they didn't know.

I asked the resident for some details about the illness, but these clinical facts only pointed to one thing—both mother and son had a viral-type pneumonia. The epidemiological facts, however, were unusual. It's very rare for an adult and a child in the same family to develop so severe a viral pneumonia. Viruses just don't have those kinds of lines in their repertoire. They might affect adults more severely than children or children more severely than adults. But for an adult and a child to be so desperately ill from a virus almost simultaneously was an act that didn't fit into ordinary Broadway plays. If it did the doctors at the medical center wouldn't have bothered to call me. This told me we were dealing with the unusual. My thinking in this direction was like pushing the button on a computer. The printout was a retrieval of my memory bank. And this particular printout had only one item on it, the only one that fit the pattern of a clustered outbreak of severe viral pneumonia.

"I think it's parrot fever."

There was silence on the other end of the phone for a few seconds and then, "What! How did you ever come up with that?"

"Easy. It's the only thing that fits."

"Come on," he said a bit arrogantly, "I don't believe it. Parrot fever! No way."

"That's my diagnosis and I plan to conduct the investigation accordingly. Did you ask if they have a parrot or some other bird in the house?"

"No, er, it didn't occur to me and they didn't say anything about it, so I guess they don't have any."

"Who's the they?" I asked him.

"Mr. Johnson. He's the father of the boy who died and the husband of Mrs. Johnson who's in the isolation unit now."

"If you didn't ask him about a bird in the home there's no way of knowing if there is or isn't one there. Just because he didn't volunteer the information is no reason to conclude they have none."

The resident's reasoning was faulty and I told him so. It's a common mistake among physicians. They assume the history for something is negative simply because the patient and relatives don't volunteer it. Remember, I'd had the same experience as a student myself presenting the history of Etta Grundig! What did he expect Mr. Johnson to say, "We have a parrot and a turtle in the yard too?" What did the Johnsons know about birds and parrot fever? Probably as much as most people, which isn't very much.

"Do me a favor and start Mrs. Johnson on high doses of antibiotics right away," I told the resident. "And if Mr. Johnson is there, have him call me right away. Oh, besides that, give me their address and telephone number at home."

He was reluctant to follow my advice, but finally agreed to do it. "Do I have to take anything?" he asked, a bit embarrassed. I almost laughed. "No you don't. It isn't spread from patients to other people, only from birds to people. But Mr. Johnson should be put on it right away because he too may have been exposed to a sick bird."

Tommie Johnson had been admitted to the medical center after his condition had deteriorated in a small suburban hospital where he spent three days. His pediatrician had originally hospitalized him because of a high fever and headache. A chest x-ray on admission showed a massive pneumonia. Tommie didn't respond to the antibiotics and his pediatrician grew worried and decided to transfer him to a larger hospital. There the antibiotics were changed, but this didn't have any effect on Tommie's condition. Two days after the transfer he died.

That same day, his mother, who had been feeling sick for a couple of days, was admitted to the large medical center with exactly the same type of pneumonia.

When I spoke to Mr. Johnson shortly after the resident called me, he said that they didn't have any birds at home. "You don't have any birds in the house?" I asked again.

"No, none at all."

"Did Tommie and your wife have any contact with any birds during the past few weeks?"

"Oh, yes," he said quickly, "with Billie."

"Who's Billie?"

"He was our parakeet. But he died. We had him for four years. A nice little feller."

Mr. Johnson was typical of many conscientious patients who answer a doctor's questions as accurately as possible—he didn't expand on the replies. He just answered whatever I asked and when he said there were no birds in the house he meant it, there weren't any. But he didn't bother to add that there had been a bird in the house because I didn't ask him that at the same time.

"When did Billie die?" I asked.

"Oh, hmm, I'd say about ten days ago, or maybe two weeks. Can't be exactly sure."

I told Mr. Johnson that I suspected that Billie the parakeet was the source of the infection that had infected his wife and son. "Can't be," he said with amazing conviction. "We had Billie for four years and he never was sick."

I questioned Mr. Johnson carefully about Billie's death. "He just got sick and died," he said. "And my wife cleaned out his cage after she buried him in the garden."

"She cleaned out the cage?"

"Yeah, it was full of dry droppings. She told me she did. She didn't want to put it down in the cellar dirty like that."

"Is that where the cage is now?"

"Yeah, I guess so, that's where she said she put it. Tommie was with her when she did because he told me when I came home from work."

"Mr. Johnson, I don't want anyone to go near that cage. Some inspectors from the Health Department will go right out to your house to pick it up and bring it in for examination. Can you meet them there?"

"Sure, I'll go right now."

Now I was absolutely sure that Mrs. Johnson was suffering from ornithosis, the scientific name for parrot fever. Mr. Johnson gave me the missing link.

The disease is caused by a microbe known as *Chlamydia psittaci*. It's an organism which is slightly bigger than a virus but smaller than most bacteria. There are various strains of this organism, some being more virulent than others. But they can all cause pneumonia in humans. This pneumonia resembles the kind caused by viruses. The organism invades the walls of the air sacs of the lungs and causes them to swell and become inflamed. As the infection progresses, the air sacs fill up with liquid and cellular debris, preventing air from getting in. The end result is that the patient can't get any oxygen into his body.

As soon as I finished speaking with Mr. Johnson, I called Todd and Latimer and told them the story. "We can bring the cage into the labs in an isolation sac," Todd said. "And we had better disinfect the area in the basement where it was stored." He and Latimer didn't think the organism could have survived anywhere else in the house. "But how about the dead parakeet buried in the garden?" I asked.

"If it had just died, we would put it in a two-percent cresol solution and then incinerate it in the lab. But since the body has been buried for almost two weeks, it's best to leave it there. The chlamydia won't survive."

Latimer and two inspectors went out to the Johnson house to pick up the cage and disinfect the cellar. But before going, they took a loading dose of tetracycline to protect themselves.

247

We tested Billie's cage at the laboratories and found it infected with *Chlamydia psittaci.* "But where did the bird get it from?" asked the chastened resident when I called to give him the results.

"He probably had it for years. Birds can act as healthy carriers for many years. The organism lives in their bodies without causing them any harm. It's not even passed in their droppings."

"So there's no way you can tell a bird has it or not if it's healthy. Is that right?"

"More or less," I told him. "You could isolate the organism from a bird that's a healthy carrier. But it wouldn't occur to people to do this."

Billie had acted as a healthy carrier and then because of either old age or because of another illness, his resistance to the organism weakened. It multiplied inside his body, caused a fulminating infection and before killing him passed out in his droppings. When Mrs. Johnson cleaned the cage, with Tommie standing nearby, she stirred up almost invisible clouds of dust particles loaded with the microbe. Once in the air, it was easy for the organism to gain access to their lungs. One shallow breath and it was on its way.

The United States Public Health Service and Department of Agriculture have been aware of the danger of ornithosis in imported birds for years. In order to protect Americans who purchase these birds they require that all imported birds be kept in quarantine for several weeks during which time they are fed seed treated with tetracycline. This antibiotic effectively kills the microbe of parrot fever in any bird which might be harboring it. Unfortunately, many exotic birds are smuggled illegally into the United States from South and Central America via Florida. They aren't subjected to quarantine and treatment with tetracycline-coated seed. And although they look healthy, they may in fact be harboring the microbe which causes lethal parrot fever. This was one of the reasons why Latimer and Todd made such an effort to confiscate smuggled birds. Also, many of these species are endangered, and their importation is prohibited. Contrary to popular belief, parrots and parakeets aren't the only birds that carry the disease. So do pigeons, ducks, chickens, pheasants and turkeys.

Mrs. Johnson was given intensive treatment for several days, but in spite of it she died. What a terrible tragedy it was. The strain

248

Billie carried was one of the most virulent and resisted the effects of the antibiotics.

When the resident first called me about Mrs. Johnson and Tommie and I stuck to my diagnosis in spite of his sharp disagreement, he commented that I was endowed with a generous supply of ego and self-confidence. He was right. But I don't think he realized that these were tempered with knowledge and experience. It was this combination which gave me the courage of my convictions, even in the face of adverse comment and disagreement from the staff of a prestigious medical center. A less seasoned man might have backed down and if he had the diagnosis would not have been made until much later on or never.

An older colleague of mine once said that the greatest proof of being a full-fledged epidemiologist is sticking to your guns, following your sensitive and highly trained instincts and resisting the intimidation of other people's opinions. In the final analysis, the epidemiologist must stand on his own two feet. To be sure, he makes mistakes and wrong guesses. But the business of medical detection is full of blind alleys and dead ends. Every time I went down a blind alley I learned something new. So while I may have been full-fledged, I was still learning all the time. It's a continuous process and I knew it would span the length of my professional career.

This was dramatically demonstrated to me in July 1976 when an unknown disease suddenly caused an explosive epidemic among people attending an American Legion convention at the Bellevue Stratford Hotel in Philadelphia. Before it was over there were 182 proven cases and 29 deaths. People were stricken with a severe pneumonia which in many ways resembles that caused by a number of viruses. But the first symptoms are much like those due to the flu—muscle aches, headache and fever. Over a dozen epidemiologists were sent to Philadelphia by the Center for Disease Control to track down what at first appeared to be an unknown killer.

Many people, including physicians, were dumbstruck by the sudden occurrence of a highly fatal disease whose cause, source and means of spread were unknown. At first some epidemiologists, and I was among them, thought that the disease might be ornithosis—parrot fever. Our reasons were that the disease in Philadelphia

249

resembled ornithosis in the way it affected individual patients. And from the epidemiological point of view it behaved in a similar fashion in that it was spread through the air and not transmitted from one person to another. That crucial piece of intelligence was uncovered early in the investigation by CDC epidemiologists. But we were wrong. When the epidemic first started, some, including epidemiologists from the Center for Disease Control, speculated that it might be swine flu. But this also proved to be wrong. No quick answers were forthcoming, but there were other theories. One of these was that the disease was due to nickel carbonyl, a poisonous gas produced by burning carbon paper. Because traces of nickel were found in the lungs of Legionnaires dying of the disease, it was theorized that the burning of carbon paper in the hotel incinerator might have produced nickel carbonyl. But this theory, like others, was rapidly discarded when experienced industrial chemists pointed out that the amount of nickel in the lung tissues of the dead Legionnaires was too high to have come from the poisonous gas. Then it was discovered that the autopsy tissues had been cut with scalpels consisting of stainless steel containing nickel.

In January 1977, the Center for Disease Control announced that its scientists had isolated a bacterium from the lungs of four of six patients who had died of the disease. These scientists had also meticulously examined these tissue samples for viruses, other bacteria, fungi and other types of microbes. But the only thing they found was a strange new bacterium. Later that year, they published a detailed description of their findings in the *New England Journal of Medicine.* This "new" bacterium was given the name *Legionella pneumophilia,* which roughly translated means "lung-loving legion." It is also known as LDB—Legionnaires' disease bacillus to epidemiologists and other medical specialists. Certainly the organism isn't new to the world. What is new is man's discovery of it, made possible by modern advances in laboratory techniques. LDB is a difficult microbe to isolate in the laboratory, requiring time, patience and skill.

During the exhaustive investigation into the Philadelphia epidemic, CDC epidemiologists came to realize that other mystery outbreaks which had occurred in the past and which had been investigated by epidemiologists were exactly like Legionnaires' disease. One of the earliest of these was in 1965 at St. Elizabeth's

Hospital in Washington, D.C. There was another in 1968 in Pontiac, Michigan. After the epidemic at the Bellevue Stratford Hotel in 1976, others were detected. Among these were an epidemic in a hospital in Burlington, Vermont, in 1977; in a hotel-student union complex in Bloomington, Indiana, in 1978; in a hospital in Memphis, Tennessee, and at the Wadsworth Veterans Administration Hospital in Los Angeles. The occurrence of these epidemics doesn't mean that the disease is increasing in frequency. In large measure it reflects the detection of epidemics which have been occurring here and there for quite some time by physicians who are now on the lookout for them. In the past, a number of epidemics went unnoticed or were thought to be outbreaks of the flu.

With each investigation, epidemiologists have come to learn a little more about Legionnaires' disease. Studies of people's blood for antibodies to the LDB demonstrate that a sizable proportion of the healthy population are positive, meaning that they have been infected at some time in the past with the microbe. They may have had a mild flulike illness or perhaps no illness at all because this microbe causes a wide spectrum of illness from very mild to lethal.

I never anticipated having any involvement with an epidemic of Legionnaires' disease. But I was wrong. In June 1978, I became professor and chairman of the Department of Preventive Medicine and Community Health at the Downstate Medical Center of the State University of New York, having resigned my position as Commissioner of Health of New York City in March of the same year. I had no way of knowing that two months later, in August, two patients would be admitted to the Kings County Hospital, which is a few feet away from my office at the medical school, and be found to have Legionnaires' disease.

But the story began at another Downstate-affiliated hospital, St. John's Episcopal, a few miles away. On August 11, a thirty-year-old man became ill with a respiratory ailment, developed a pneumonia and was admitted to the hospital. He died there on August 25, in spite of the heroic efforts to save him. The day before he died, on August 24, two of his brothers were admitted to Kings County Hospital suffering from the same disease. Both of them had gotten ill around the twentieth of August.

Dr. Felix Taubman, the director of the Department of Medicine at St. John's, suspected all along that his patient had Legionnaires'

251

disease. And at Kings County, the same diagnosis was made in the two brothers by Dr. Ellie Goldstein, an infectious-disease specialist. Dr. Goldstein had been involved in the epidemic of Legionnaires' disease at the Wadsworth Veterans Administration Hospital in California and had a great deal of experience with the illness. When the two brothers told him that their brother was at St. John's Episcopal Hospital, he contacted Dr. Taubman. They both realized that they had unearthed an outbreak. But they didn't have any idea how big it was, whom it was affecting, nor where it was centered. All three brothers lived in the same neighborhood in Brooklyn. Was that the site of the epidemic? Possibly. But all of them also worked in the same part of Manhattan—the garment center. That also was clearly a possibility. They informed Dr. John Marr, my successor as New York City's chief epidemiologist. Dr. Marr was initially stumped like Goldstein and Taubman. Where did they contract it?, they all asked. But then on September 1, physicians at Bellevue Hospital called Dr. Marr to tell him that a forty-four-year-old man had been hospitalized with what they thought was Legionnaires' disease. He worked in the garment center. But what was significant was that he didn't live in Brooklyn but worked in precisely the same small section of the garment center as the three brothers from Brooklyn. It was obvious now that the epidemic was in the garment center.

Dr. Marr concentrated his investigation in the area where the patients worked—West 35th Street between Broadway and Seventh Avenue. On September 5, blood specimens were taken from the workers in the building where the two surviving brothers from Brooklyn worked. And epidemiologists interviewed the workers in order to find out if they had been ill. They learned that seventeen of thirty workers (57 percent) had been ill with fever, cough, weakness and headache in middle-to-late August. This information plus subsequent laboratory studies rapidly pinpointed this block as the epicenter of the epidemic.

That evening the public was told of the epidemic for the first time. Here was a new disease, unknown to most, but known to be fatal in some, caused by a recently discovered microbe and transmitted in a way unknown even to experts, smack in the center of the city. Panic and alarm swept the city. Mayor Koch and the city's health officials did their best to calm people's fears and launched a massive effort to uncover the source of the epidemic. Dr. David Fraser of the CDC, a leading authority on the disease, came to assist in the investigation as did Dr. William Foege, the director of the Center for Disease Control.

A special Task Force was formed, headed by a deputy mayor. They ordered the streets cleaned and washed and had the subway stations hosed down in an attempt to destroy *Legionella pneumophilia*, the tiny rodlike microbe which everyone knew was around, but which no one could find. Where was it? Where did it come from? How did it get here? No one knew the answers to these questions. As I witnessed these efforts on the evening television news broadcast, I was reminded of Africa, of the *imam's* magic water containing dissolved Arabic letters from the Koran, of talismans and charms and of garlic from the Middle Ages. I reflected on what I saw even while many of my colleagues laughed. For here was technological man face to face with the unknown and his response was no different from so-called primitive man's.

It is difficult to conduct a meticulous epidemiological investigation in the public glare and while beset with demands that miracles be performed to stop the epidemic. But the epidemiologists whose task it was to deal with this epidemic proceeded with their work and within a few days produced sufficient data to characterize it. Dr. Marr called me and asked my advice about how to go forward with certain aspects of the investigation. And then a few days later, my successor as Commissioner of Health, Dr. Reinaldo Ferrer, set up a Legionnaires' Disease Advisory Committee, composed of epidemiologists and other public-health experts. I was a member of the committee.

The committee met on September 11 and was briefed by both Dr. Fraser of the CDC and by Dr. Marr. A total of forty-one persons had been hospitalized with the disease. Of these three died. The last case had occurred only the day before, but from the data it appeared that the epidemic had reached its peak during the latter part of August. Members of the committee voiced concern about water towers and central air-conditioning units in the area as these have been found to be the source of other epidemics of Legionnaires' disease. On the basis of what is known to date, it appears that the LDB can thrive in the slime that often accumulates in these units.

Public furor and interest gradually declined as it became apparent that no further cases were occurring and epidemiologists were able to proceed with their investigation. They came up with some surprising findings. On examining the blood of 884 garment-center workers, they found that 24.3 percent had antibodies to the microbe. By comparison 16.0 percent of 244 workers in the Bronx and 24.8 percent of 246 workers in another area of Manhattan had antibodies. This data suggests that Legionnaires' disease has been around the city for quite some time. There were a total of fifty-seven cases of the disease during the August epidemic, more than half of them clustered around work locations on West 35th Street between Seventh Avenue and Broadway. Most who contracted the disease worked outdoors at such jobs as pushing clothes racks along the streets. This strongly suggests that the disease was contracted on the street and not inside buildings. The scientific consensus, based on blood studies of healthy people and on the investigations of epidemics, is that Legionnaires' disease is fairly ubiquitous. But for reasons not yet fully understood it occasionally causes serious explosive epidemics.

On January 12, 1979, the *New York Times* carried a frontpage story reporting that the bacterium that causes Legionnaires' disease was isolated from water samples taken from an air-conditioning water-cooling tower atop Macy's Department Store which overlooks the West 35th Street area where the disease had broken out. I was interviewed by the *New York Times* the day before when I first learned of this finding at the second meeting of the Legionnaires' Disease Advisory Committee. The *Times* asked me if I thought that the water in the tower was the source of the epidemic. I replied that the index of suspicion was very high because the tower in question was located directly across the street from where so many of the cases occurred.

Water in towers of this kind is circulated on the outside of rooftop air-conditioning units in order to cool them down. The water doesn't get into the ducts of the air-conditioning system, but it is transformed into a spray on the roof as it cascades down the exterior of the unit. This spray, according to one epidemiologist who visited the roof during the investigation, fell down onto West 35th Street below.

Two weeks after the *New York Times* story, the Department of

Health announced that the bacterium had been isolated from a second water tower on Macy's roof. In both instances the water samples were taken during the epidemic investigations and after that, Macy's stated in the *Times*, they drained, cleaned and disinfected the units.

The epidemic aroused great interest within the Downstate community of hospitals not only because three of the patients were hospitalized in them, but more importantly because two members of the faculty, Taubman and Goldstein, were responsible for uncovering the existence of the epidemic. It took unusual ability to diagnose Legionnaires' disease in the first place, and even more to establish the fact that an outbreak had taken place. The Department of Medicine decided to devote one of its Grand Rounds to a discussion of Legionnaires' disease and a few months later the Department of Pediatrics did the same. I was invited to discuss the epidemiology of the disease in the garment center. As I prepared my presentation, I thought back eighteen years to the time I presented Mrs. Grundig's case at Grand Rounds and produced a long list of exotic and improbable diagnoses. And now I was discussing one of the most unusual diseases known to man. Numerous questions followed and many people wanted a concise yes or no answer to "Were the towers on Macy's roof the source of the bacterium which caused the epidemic?" I couldn't give them a yes or no answer. True the organisms were found there and true the towers and the spray they generated were across the street from where so many became ill, but this wasn't absolute proof. For the real source could have been another tower on another building in the neighborhood. Whether the presence of the Legionnaires' disease bacillus in the towers and the epidemic are related in a cause-and-effect fashion or are only coincidental to one another remains an unanswered question.

CHAPTER 21

FROM EPIDEMIOLOGIST
TO ADMINISTRATOR

As summer rolled around again, Bill Herbert completed his two years with the Epidemic Intelligence Service and went out West to start his residency training in internal medicine. He was a splendid epidemiologist with a remarkable track record of experience and achievement and I was sorry to see him leave. In a sense he was putting most of this behind because he was entering a specialty where he would have little opportunity to use his epidemiologic skills and knowledge. For him, as for most, epidemiology was a chapter in his career, a rich and rewarding moment, but fleeting. I was saddened by his departure not only because it meant the loss of a trusted colleague whose competence and knowledge I respected, but also because of what his departure symbolized. All over the country, young physicians like Bill were leaving their positions with the Epidemic Intelligence Service and going into other specialties of medicine.

When they did leave, their unique training, experience and medical detection skills were shelved, filed away like a high-school yearbook and eventually remembered only occasionally with the passage of time. Epidemiology wasn't able to hold them because the disadvantages attached to it were too great. Most young epidemiologists come to realize as Bill did that a career in communicable-disease epidemiology meant working in public service for low salaries, with shrinking budgets, ever-increasing frustrations and mounting bureaucratic responsibilities. After a while, these negative characteristics begin to outweigh the rewards and challenges epidemiology has to offer. Young physicians are willing to sacrifice for a while, but not for a lifetime.

I loved epidemiology and enjoyed being New York City's top medical detective. Milton Helpern, who was then the Chief Medical Examiner of New York City, and I often said that we had the two most interesting medical jobs in the city. While my task was to detect the source and mode of spread of infections and stamp them out in order to save lives, his was to detect the real cause and manner of death in order to bring those responsible to justice. In a sense we were both medical detectives, but of a different sort. Milt Helpern and I worked on a number of problems together and after his death I became a trustee of the Milton Helpern Library of Legal Medicine which was established in his honor.

I shared my concerns with Milt and he was understanding. He too had difficulty in recruiting young pathologists into his department, even though the work was fascinating. The reasons were the same—low salaries, shrinking budgets and increasing frustration. I came to realize that a full-time career in epidemiology would demand a level of personal sacrifice which I just couldn't make. I didn't share these nagging doubts with my staff, but more and more they occupied my mind.

"That's the way it goes," Murray said the day Bill left. "They come and they go, and me, well, I just stay on and watch the parade."

Soon after Bill left, the Center for Disease Control asked me to go to India for a few weeks as an advisor on the massive effort then being made to eradicate smallpox from its last earthly bastion. I accepted and planned to leave in January of 1974, using up some of the two months of vacation time I had accumulated. I saw the trip as a chance to get away and think, to rethink my future career and to arrive at a decision that so far was the hardest I had ever faced. But other events changed all these plans.

In November I went to Houston to attend the annual meeting of the American Society of Tropical Medicine and Hygiene. There I

258

met a young physician who was completing his U.S. Army service. Dr. John Marr was a graduate of Yale and the New York Medical College, and had already completed his training in both internal medicine and public health. His training was almost identical to mine and we both shared a keen interest in tropical medicine. He very much wanted to return to New York City and begin a career as an epidemiologist. What a rare find he was! After the meeting I stayed in close contact with him and kept him informed about my plans for reorganizing the bureau and training the public-health nurses as epidemiologists. I offered him a position as a full-time epidemiologist and he accepted.

As 1973 drew to a close a mayoral election took place in New York City. Abraham D. Beame, then the city comptroller, was elected. Mayoral elections didn't affect the professional staff of the Department of Health since the positions they held were nonpolitical. And not infrequently, newly elected mayors didn't change the top executives of the department. But at the time of the election, no one knew for sure what Mayor-elect Beame would do. During his campaign he promised to reprofessionalize the Department of Health, alluding to the policies of his predecessor, Mayor John V. Lindsay. During the late 1960s there was a general countrywide shift in public-health administration to replace physicians in executive positions with lay administrators trained in sophisticated management techniques. Under Lindsay, the Department of Health was in the forefront of this movement. But by 1973 it was clear that the experiment was a dismal failure. Managers and fiscal experts were no more adept at dealing with the insurmountable health problems of the city than their physician predecessors had been. In fact their performance was much worse because they lacked medical skills and medical knowledge. Under their stewardship the department went on the skids. The largest health department in the nation was no longer viewed as a model.

As the Director of the Bureau of Infectious Disease Control I was constantly exposed to the never-ending deluge of confusing and conflicting so-called managerial reforms initiated by this executive team of people who didn't have the credentials to manage. But the bureau dealt with such complex and highly technical problems beyond their comprehension that I was able to fend off their

259

incursions with relative ease. It was a wearing and tiring game and it was being played not only in New York City but all over the country.

Mayor Beame set up a search committee to find a new Commissioner of Health. Among the leaders of this committee was Dr. Howard A. Rusk, founder of the Institute of Rehabilitation Medicine at New York University Medical Center, and Dr. John Knowles, president of the Rockefeller Foundation. Dr. Rusk had always been a strong force in public-health affairs in the city and his views were respected by Mayor Beame as they were by many other mayors before. And John Knowles, who at a very young age became the director of the prestigious Massachusetts General Hospital, was one of the leading health administrators in the country. They and the other members of the committee recommended that Dr. Lowell E. Bellin be appointed Commissioner of Health. And on January 7, 1974, Mayor Beame officially made the announcement.

Dr. Bellin had left the department (shortly after he hired me) to become professor and chairman of the Department of Public Health Administration at the Columbia University School of Public Health.

A few days after his return to the Health Department, Ida Peters came rushing into my office saying, "The Commissioner wants you in his office immediately!"

I had no idea why he wanted to see me. Word had reached me though that he had summoned other bureau directors and executive and managerial personnel and had been very candid about his perceptions of their past performance. Some realized that they would have to find other jobs. So when I took the elevator to go up to his temporary sixth-floor office it was with considerable trepidation. How did I know what people might have told him about me? I had been around bureaucracies long enough to know that the reality presented to a boss wasn't always reality. My crusade to change the bureau had earned me a fair share of enemies.

When I walked into the office he asked me to sit down at the large oak conference table which dominated the center of the room. He sat himself directly opposite me. We hadn't seen one another in almost two years and he struck me as being extremely intense and formal compared with when I first met him. I sensed he had something important to tell me.

Leaning over the table he said, "I've heard all about what you've been doing in the bureau the past two years."

My heart was pounding. Thoughts flashed through my mind. The union, the part-time doctors, the veterinarians, the clerical staff—none of them were too happy with my planned changes. What did Bellin know about them and more importantly how did he feel about them?

I was almost sure he was going to fire me.

Then he hit me with a bolt of lightning. "I want you to be the First Deputy Health Commissioner."

I was dumbstruck. I stared at him in disbelief. He stared back. "Me?"

"Yes, you, and I'll tell you why," he said. "Anyone who spent five years in Africa fighting cholera and smallpox has something extra special about him. And you've done a fantastic job in the Bureau of Infectious Disease Control." He smiled. "I've heard all about it. Not too many would have had the courage to stick through it the way you have. Now, is that reason enough?"

As he spoke I knew I would have to give him an answer right away. He wasn't a man who was tolerant of indecision. He respected decisions made with speed, confidence, certitude. This was an enormous one and I had to make it now.

"As First Deputy," he went on, "you'll be running the department on a day-to-day basis. In effect you'll be the Commissioner of Health. I have to devote a lot of my time to the Health and Hospitals Corporation since I'm Chairman of the Board."

A lot of mixed feelings churned inside me. If I accepted it might mean leaving epidemiology permanently. I who always lamented the departure of so many other good physicians from the field would be doing the same thing myself. Until that morning I hadn't made my own internal decision yet about epidemiology. Bellin's offer embodied not just the prospect of a new career but also a call for me to decide right then and there about my future in epidemiology. While we looked at one another across the table a scene flashed through my mind from twenty years before. It was the day I met with Mr. Wright at the American Museum of Natural Histo-

261

ry. And although my career had been fashioned according to the advice he gave me that January day, somehow his words had been lost in my subconscious over time. They now came back to me in this crucial moment—"If you become a physician, you can also be an anthropologist, a naturalist, whatever else you want to be . . ." So Bellin's offer didn't represent an all or none choice. It didn't mean closing my interest in epidemiology completely. But it required rearranging it in my professional life, and that I was willing to do.

My experience in epidemiology had so far been fulfilling and gratifying. My reorganization plans for the bureau were well on their way to being implemented. I thought and pondered. I knew as did everyone in the department that the First Deputy Commissioner often became the next Commissioner of Health. All of this loomed in front of me like an enormous challenge and I felt the excitement of an explorer moving into an unknown world, the kind of excitement I felt when I first landed in Nairobi, when I walked the plains of Tanganyika with Kambaragi, when I set off for Titilan.

Here was a chance to expand my skills and experience in the broader fields of public health and administration in a city with the most complex and overwhelming health-care problems in the country. But I was apprehensive about assuming these enormous responsibilities, because I had never had any prior experience with them. I had no way of knowing at the time how much I would be able to draw upon my previous training and expertise as a medical detective. In a reality which was still in the future, epidemiology would play an important part. I reflected for a few seconds and then decided. "I accept." With those two words I launched myself into a new adventure.

"You had better find a replacement for yourself," Bellin said as I started for the door.

"I already have," I said smiling back. "He's down in Houston."

"You see," he replied, "you're a natural administrator."

Index

265

269

271